SEATED
TAIJI AND
QIGONG

of related interest

Chair Yoga
Seated Exercises for Health and Wellbeing
Edeltraud Rohnfeld
Illustrated by Edeltraud Rohnfeld
ISBN 978 1 84819 078 8
eISBN 978 0 85701 056 8

Qigong for Multiple Sclerosis
Finding Your Feet Again
Nigel Mills
ISBN 978 1 84819 019 1
eISBN 978 0 85701 029 2

Managing Depression with Qigong
Frances Gaik
ISBN 978 1 84819 018 4
eISBN 978 0 85701 029 2

Managing Stress with Qigong
Gordon Faulkner
Foreword by Carole Bridge
ISBN 978 1 84819 035 1
eISBN 978 0 85701 016 2

Curves, Twists and Bends
A Practical Guide to Pilates for Scoliosis
Annette Wellings and Alan Herdman
ISBN 978 1 84819 025 2
eISBN 978 0 85701 009 4

Chi for Children
A Practical Guide to Teaching Tai Chi and Qigong in Schools and the Community
Betty Sutherland
ISBN 978 1 84819 055 9

SEATED
TAIJI AND
QIGONG

Guided Therapeutic Exercises to Manage
Stress and Balance Mind, Body and Spirit

Cynthia W. Quarta

Foreword by Michelle Maloney Vallie, LCPC, LAC, PhD

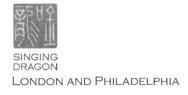

SINGING
DRAGON
LONDON AND PHILADELPHIA

First published in 2012
by Singing Dragon
an imprint of Jessica Kingsley Publishers
116 Pentonville Road
London N1 9JB, UK
and
400 Market Street, Suite 400
Philadelphia, PA 19106, USA

www.singingdragon.com

Library of Congress Cataloging in Publication Data
A CIP catalog record for this book is available from the Library of Congress

British Library Cataloguing in Publication Data
A CIP catalogue record for this book is available from the British Library

ISBN 978 1 84819 088 7
eISBN 978 0 85701 071 1

Printed and bound in Great Britain

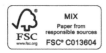

To my family for their continuing support and to my students who have given me more than I can ever repay

CONTENTS

FOREWORD

There should be no contention that stress in the Western world is almost epidemic, and, despite our attempts to control and seize it, it seems to control us and threaten our well-being. As health professionals, we know that often the clients who are seeking help are struggling with managing the incessant demands of their jobs and their families in addition to their physical illnesses or limitations. In their strivings to heal in a myriad of ways, clients paradoxically place many expectations on themselves to improve and to achieve more, rather than stopping a moment to appreciate what they have accomplished and examine what they may glean from their life's journeys. Despite our clients' physical illnesses or attempts at rehabilitation, we as professionals are in great need of quality resources to aid clients in managing their stress. In so doing, clients can enjoy greater benefits from their rehabilitation for both healthier bodies and healthier minds.

John Ciardi eloquently spoke of our common stress illness in this way:

> an ulcer is an unkissed imagination taking its revenge for having been jilted. It is an undanced dance, an unpainted watercolor, an unwritten poem. It is a sign that a clear spring of joy has not been tapped and must break through, muddily, on its own.[1]

But let's not teach clients to treat this spring of wellness as yet another frantic goal to be obtained; better yet, let us convey that it is acceptable to live on the edge of possibility, the other side of language, the other side of ego, enjoying the process of their strivings, not their products.

All of this advice sounds good, but how can we really help clients live in their demanding worlds while gaining a healthier, more joyful perspective for their bodies and minds? I am confident that this book will provide many of the answers for health professionals. Through modified Taiji and Qigong methods, reducing stress is now simpler and easier to teach and to understand. Although

---

1 Quote attributed to a speech given by John Ciardi to a group of business people. For a comprehensive collection of the works of John Ciardi, contact the University of Arkansas, Fayetteville, AR 72701, USA.

the stress in all of our lives will not disappear, we hope that your clients will be inspired to dance, paint, write, work, study, or enjoy any of their chosen endeavors with less stress, more energy, an enlivened physical body, and a greater appreciation for their travels through life, rather than their destinations.

Michelle Maloney Vallie, LCPC, LAC, PhD
Outpatient Therapist, Great Falls, Montana, Center for Mental Health

Introduction

I first developed a system of seated Taiji exercises while employed as program supervisor at a local retirement community. At that time, I had been studying and teaching dance and martial arts for many years. When I first began my job as program supervisor, the residents of the retirement community required little or no assistance with their daily activities and so, with a few adjustments, I was able to use much of my training to lead a daily exercise class.

When the facility changed from one for independent seniors to an exclusively assisted-living community, I had to re-evaluate the entire activities program. Many of the standard activities were age- and condition-appropriate even for those who were dependent on walkers, canes, or wheelchairs. Our exercise class, however, needed extensive revision! My challenge was to find exercises that accommodated all of the participants: those who were able to stand, those who could stand but relied on walkers, and those who were confined to wheelchairs, unable to stand at all.

Most importantly, this new exercise program had to be designed in such a way that strengthening, flexibility, improved circulation, and so on were not lost as a result of the necessary modifications. With the help of many wonderful and involved residents, I created an exercise program that resulted in dramatic changes in the health and fitness level of the participants. Since that time, I've had the opportunity to teach the same program—standing and seated—to many different age groups.

I now teach middle-aged adults and college students who are of both traditional and non-traditional age and I've recently added Qigong exercises as the "warm-up" period of the class. As a result, I have discovered another dimension to the benefits of practicing the type of exercise and wellness systems developed in China centuries ago. My students and I agree that Taiji and Qigong by themselves or in combination are useful in clearing the mind and in preparing them for writing papers, studying difficult subjects, and taking exams. This addition has proven of great benefit to the overall effectiveness of the exercises, particularly in terms of alleviating stress.

Entering college right out of high school presents special challenges: being away from home, adjusting to the demands of college level classes, and maintaining the necessary GPA (grade point average) to remain in school. One of my young college students tells me that she performs the entire Yang short form or a set of Qigong exercises before taking exams rather than reviewing the material. She knows the subject matter but has had difficulty in the past when faced with test questions. Now, she has a way to clear her mind and relax. Her stress level is down and her grades have improved.

Students striving to attain a degree later in life are often juggling children, spouses, a part- or full-time job, the strain of attending classes, writing papers, and taking exams. Each and every one of these students has praised the benefits of Taiji and Qigong in relieving the fatigue and stress in their busy lives. A former Taiji student of non-traditional age, who now serves as an advisor to incoming students, recommends the use of breathing exercises to these new students in order to improve their performance on tests and to clear their minds before writing papers.

Whatever level of patient you, as a health care professional, are dealing with, you are certainly aware of the stresses that modern life, advanced age, chronic illness, disability, or a post-surgical period can place on your patients. Dealing with illness and disease every day places stress on you as well. While moderate levels of stress may drive us to greater productivity, excessive stress can sink us into sickness and depression.

1

CHINESE MEDICINE

There are 11 famous Chinese medical books that have survived from ancient times. These are the *Yellow Emperor's Classic of Medicine*, the *Divine Husbandman's Classic of Materia Medica*, the *Classic of Difficult Issues*, the *Treatise on Febrile Diseases*, the *Synopsis of the Golden Cabinet*, the *Systematic Classic of Acupuncture and Moxibustion*, the *Grand Materia Medica*, the *Pulse Classic*, the *Systematic Differentiation of Warm Diseases*, *Tang Materia Medica*, and *Master Hua's Classic of the Central Viscera*.

The *Yellow Emperor's Classic of Medicine* is still in use today in some medical schools in Europe, Asia, and the United States. This Chinese classic lays out the foundations of traditional Chinese medicine (TCM): the theory of balance (*yin/yang*), the five elements, the concept of holism, and a description of the meridians, organs, emotions, and pathogens. Topics are discussed in dialogue format between the Yellow Emperor and a physician, Qi Bo. Eighty-one chapters deal with general health questions and cover areas of a spiritual nature such as the unity of human nature and nature, as well as the interaction between human beings and the environment.

The *Divine Husbandman's Classic of Materia Medica* is concerned with a description of herbs and their uses. It discusses 365 herbs, their functions, and clinical applications, and provides a classification of superior, middle, and inferior herbs.

The *Classic of Difficult Issues* takes the subjects discussed in the *Yellow Emperor's Classic of Medicine* a step further by explaining the relationship of the dynamics of *qi* in human physiology, an identification of acupuncture points, and the use of pulse points in diagnosing illness.

Diseases that involve fevers are addressed in the medical classic, the *Treatise on Febrile Diseases*. Zhang Zhongjing describes 113 treatments for patients presenting with severe and long-term fevers. The treatments are designed to address such diverse diseases as the common cold and liver cancer.

The *Synopsis of the Golden Cabinet* not only describes gynecological disorders, internal diseases, and dermatological conditions, but also lays out a comprehensive system for dealing with each of these complaints.

As the title implies, the *Systematic Classic of Acupuncture and Moxibustion* describes all the acupuncture points in use at the time of its publication (around 282 AD). Moxibustion refers to the use of heat to relieve pain.

Diagnosis under the TCM system involves the reading of pulse points throughout the body. Illnesses are identified by a comparison between the various pulse points. In this book, 24 pulse points are defined in diagnostic and prognostic terms. The patient's symptoms, together with a reading of each of the pulse points, guide the physician in his/her choice of treatments.

Almost a thousand years after the publication of the first medical classic dealing with the use of herbs, an updated version was written by Su Jing. Called either the *Newly Revised Materia Medica* or the *Tang Materia Medica* because it was published during the Tang Dynasty, this treatise contains excellent illustrations of 844 herbs. Information on the names, uses, decoctions, and methods of collections of each of these herbs is also discussed in the *Newly Revised Materia Medica*. Herbs are divided into groups such as minerals, grasses, animals, fish, fruits, vegetables, and so on.

The most famous physician in the history of China is Hua Tuo who practiced medicine during the latter part of the Han Dynasty. His book, *Master Hua's Classic of the Central Viscera*, is the oldest known treatise of internal medicine in the world. Hua Tuo describes formulae for concocting herbs for use in anesthetizing a patient during surgery. It is important to note that acupuncture was also used for this purpose and is still in use today for both medical and dental surgeries. Most importantly for us, Dr. Hua Tuo also created perhaps the first Qigong form, which he called the "five animal forms."

Chinese medicine makes use of the same principles that apply to the actions and relationships of the five elements to diagnose and treat ailments of the human body. Each of the organs of the body is either a *yin* organ or a *yang* organ. There are five *yang* or empty organs and six *yin* or solid organs. The small and large intestines, the stomach, the bladder, and the gallbladder are the male, or empty, organs of the body. The *yin* organs are the lungs, the kidneys, the liver, the spleen, and the heart.

In addition, each of these organs reflects the characteristics of one of the five basic elements found in nature. The heart (*yin*) and the small intestine (*yang*) are represented by fire. The element that douses fire is water and represents the kidneys (*yin*) and the bladder (*yang*). That which fire destroys or alters is metal and is associated with the lungs (*yin*) and the large intestine (*yang*). Metals are retrieved from the earth and earth is associated with the spleen (*yin*) and the stomach (*yang*). Wood or trees grow in the earth and wood relates in Chinese medicine to the liver (*yin*) and the gallbladder (*yang*). The sixth *yin* organ is composed of those parts of the body that are sensory organs: the eyes, tongue, mouth, nose, and ears. Each of these sensory organs relates to a different element. The eyes are associated with wood, the tongue with fire, the mouth with earth, the nose with metal, and the ears with water.

Rather than treat only the diseased organ as is the procedure in Western medicine, a Chinese medical practitioner treats the organ's opposite with equal care and attention. To put it simply, a problem with the patient's liver may involve the treatment of the gallbladder because the source of the illness may be the result of a weakness on the part of the gallbladder rather than the liver itself. Conversely, weakness of the liver may cause disease in the gallbladder or in some other related organ.

The importance of balancing the *yin* and the *yang* is paramount in the treatment of human ailments as well. A patient who suffers from the cold will receive herbs that warm the blood, exercises, and acupuncture treatments to promote better circulation, and perhaps a diet that is high in protein.

Because the Chinese approach to wellness is a *holistic* one, further attention is given to the proper dynamic balance between the physical, spiritual, and mental state of each patient. Disease is not considered to be purely one of a specific physical ailment but also one that affects or is affected by the patient's frame of mind and level of spiritual awareness. Therefore, it is essential to balance the body, mind, and spirit in order to return the patient to a state of wholeness and well-being using the five elements, belief in invisible pathways called meridians, and the three *dan tians* as the basis for a variety of treatments. That which constitutes the healing energy stored in those *dan tians* and identified as the *Three Treasures* is called *qi*.

The *qi* of Taiji and Qigong

If we define *qi* as "energy," we can then begin to understand the term in relationship to the movements of both Taiji and Qigong. The movements in both these exercise forms, and more importantly the mind-directed flow of this energy, are designed with the express purpose of releasing that energy from the *dan tians* in which it is stored. If properly practiced, both exercises will allow the *qi* to "sink deeply and settle into the bones."

The concept of *qi* is at the very center of Chinese philosophy. According to Wolfgang Metzger in *Taiji Chu'an and Qigong: Techniques and Training*, this connection can be understood in four ways:

- Each human being has inherited a certain quality of *qi* that can be very high but also very low. This inherited, or prenatal, *qi* is called **Yuan Qi**.

- *Qi* is also given to us through food, the **Gu Qi** or food *qi*.

- The **Kong Qi** reaches our body through breathing and—together with the **Yuan Qi** and the **Gu Qi**—combines to form the overall *qi* or **Zheng Qi**.

- **Zheng Qi** is the all-encompassing term for several types of *qi* that have very special functions.

In addition, *qi* itself—**Zheng Qi**—has five basic functions. First, no movement of the body would be possible without *qi*. Second, *qi* provides immunity to the system from all outside pathogens. The third action of *qi* is the regulation of the conversions that take place in the body such as the change of those nutrients to blood and urine whenever we ingest food. Fourth, *qi* ensures protection from all assaults on bodily substances and organs, internal or external. Finally, *qi* regulates body temperature, ensuring sufficient blood flow for warmth in the winter and for cooling our body temperature in the summer.

The five elements

Wuxing means "five elements" in Chinese, *wu* meaning "five" and *xing*, "elements." In the West, we consider these elements—fire, wood, water, earth, and metal—to be static, inactive matter. Not so in Eastern philosophy. The Chinese Naturalist School developed the theory of the five elements more than two thousand years ago based on the premise that these elements were an integral part of the dynamic processes of nature. Further, the elements provided a system by which changes in nature could be described and natural phenomena could be classified.

The *Yinyangjia* (Naturalist School) noted the interrelationships between these elements and categorized those relationships as mutual creation, mutual closeness, mutual destruction, and mutual fear. Their mutual creation is described below:

Wood	creates	Fire
Fire	creates	Earth
Earth	creates	Metal
Metal	creates	Water
Water	creates	Wood

Each of the pairs of elements above is additionally related to another through the principle of mutual closeness. For example, wood depends upon water for its growth, and earth relies on fire because the ashes from fire replenish the earth by becoming part of the soil. Reading from left to right, the relationship between any pair of elements is one of creation. Reading from right to left indicates the pairing of the elements in terms of their mutual closeness.

In the same way, the principles of destruction and fear produce a pairing:

Wood	destroys	Earth
Earth	destroys	Water
Water	destroys	Fire
Fire	destroys	Metal
Metal	destroys	Wood

Once again, the left-to-right pairing indicates the principle of destruction or limitation. The right-to-left pairing shows the principle of fear. For example, reading from left to right, we can conclude that wood weakens or destroys earth. Wood does this by drawing nutrients from the earth for its own growth. Reading right to left, we see, then, that earth fears wood as the source of its depletion. In the same way, wood fears metal because tools made from metal are used to chop down trees, and so on.

Creation and closeness are constructive principles and are therefore activities of *yang*. Destruction and fear, on the other hand, are considered to be activities that are characteristic of *yin*.

The eight meridians

In order to be able to visualize the movement of energy through the body as we do in all the exercises described in this book, we need to know what routes we wish the energy to take. That, in turn, depends on which part of the body we are targeting and what we hope to accomplish. In this book, we will concentrate only on the eight extraordinary or vessel meridians rather than trying to keep track of all 20 energy pathways. The eight extraordinary meridians are listed below:

1. The *du mai* begins at the perineum, rises up the back and along the centerline of the body, over the scalp, down the forehead, ending at the upper palate of the mouth behind the teeth.

2. From the tip of the tongue, the *ren mai* moves down the centerline of the front of the body and back to the perineum.

3. The *chong mai* is a line that begins at the perineum and runs vertically through the three *dan tian* points.

4. The *dai mai* resembles a belt encircling the waist, starting and ending at the navel.

5. Beginning at a point on the *du mai* at about the middle of the upper back, the *yang wei mai* traverses the back of each arm and through the inside of the middle finger. *Yang wei mai* ends at the *laogong* point on the palm of the hand. When you curl your fingers, the *laogong* point is where your middle finger rests against the palm.

6. The *yin wei mai* meridian begins at the *laogong* points, traveling up the inside of each arm, across the pectoral muscles, and through the nipples. *Yin wei mai* ends at the *ren mai* before traveling a short distance along the *dai mai*.

7. Beginning at the perineum and traveling along the front of each leg are the pathways called the *yang qiao mai*. These meridians run the full length of the leg through the instep to the sole of the foot.

8. From the soles of the feet, the *yin qiao mai* moves up the inside of each foot, looping around the ankles and returning to the perineum by way of the inner thighs.

The junction points

Impediments to the natural flow of energy are most likely to occur at the junction points. For that reason, it is important to learn where these points are and to give them special attention while leading the exercises and directing your patient in the use of acupressure. As a professional dealing particularly with the elderly or disabled, it is vital that you understand these processes so that you can guide your class or patient's attention to these crucial areas.

At a point between the legs and halfway from the genitals to the anus is the junction of the *yang wei mai*, the *yin qiao mai*, the *ren mai*, the *du mai*, and the *chong mai*. This is called the *huiyin*. *Mingmen* is at a point on the *du mai* directly behind the navel. At a point along the *du mai* between the shoulder and behind the heart is the *gaohuang*. This junction point is key to the health of the heart and lungs. In the middle of the top of the head is a point called the *niyuan* that connects the *chong mai* with the *du mai*. The *laogong*, you may recall from the meridian list, is that spot on our palm where the middle finger rests when we curl our fingers. This is the point at which the *yang wei mai* and the *yin wei mai* meet. The navel itself is called *shenque* and is the junction point for the *ren mai* and the *dai mai*. The seventh junction point is called the *yongquan* and is on the sole of each foot about two-thirds of the way between the heel and the middle toe. This is the point at which the *yang qiao mai* meets the *yin qiao mai*.

Don't allow the Chinese names of these junction points and meridians to confuse you or your patients. It isn't necessary to memorize the names or worry about how to pronounce them. The important thing to keep in mind as you lead the exercises is approximately where the meridians and the junction points are located so that you can draw attention to a particular area or pathway. For example, the exercise *Bird's Feathered Hand* involves the use of the arms and hands only. You will need, then, to draw attention to the meridian that runs down the outside of the arm through the middle finger, the junction point *laogong*, and the meridian on the inside of the arm that returns the energy back to the shoulder and trunk. The exercise called *An*, however, requires a twist of the waist. In that case, you and your patients will need to add the meridian that circles the waist (the *dai mai*) to your list of targeted pathways. A diagram of all the meridians and junction points can be found in Appendix B. Use these diagrams to help you identify and point out the appropriate areas of the body as you direct your patients through the exercises.

The Three Treasures

The ancient Chinese believed that those who develop the proper balance between mind, body, and breath are in possession of *Three Treasures*. Those treasures are named *jing*, *qi*, and *shen*. They can be found in three specific locations in the body called the *dan tians*. The lower *dan tian*, discussed in the following section, is believed to be the repository for *jing*, the middle *dan tian* for *qi*, and the upper *dan tian* for *shen*. *Jing* refers to the energy or *qi* as expressed through movement or the energy produced by the body when used against an opponent. The *qi* of the middle *dan tian* denotes the "breath" of the body that is believed to reside in the middle *dan tian* in the area of the diaphragm, lungs, and solar plexus.

Superficially, *jing* is identified with the sex organs—a man's sperm and testosterone, and a woman's ovaries and estrogen. Yet, the proper definition of this term includes the entire endocrine system and all of the chemical interactions of metabolism. *Jing* is our biochemical makeup. How we grow and develop, the strength or weakness of our constitution, how we age, and whether our body retains its youthful vigor or begins to deteriorate in middle age depends on the quantity of *jing* available in the body. This is not necessarily, however, a pre-existing condition but rather is affected by the way we live our lives.

Qi resides in the middle *dan tian* (located in the solar plexus) and is most accurately defined as the functional energy of the body. Together with *jing*, it regulates maturation and aging. *Qi* is believed to be responsible for the involuntary functions of the body such as breathing and heartbeat, as well as voluntary muscle activity. *Qi* also controls the circulation, particularly the amount of oxygen in the blood and the processes of the nervous system.

Shen is associated with mental activity. Decision making, academic achievements, analytical thought, and impulse control all fall within the purview of *shen*. When expanded through meditation and concentrated effort, *shen* takes on a higher aspect related to intuition, creativity, and spirituality. Because you and your patients will be concentrating your efforts and your minds on the three *dan tians* in the Taiji exercises, the properties or treasures that reside in these locations will be activated.

The three dan tians

The three *dan tians* that house the *Three Treasures*, then, are the cultivation points from which all energy flows. The lower *dan tian* is located between the pubic bone and the navel about midway through the body, connected in Chinese medicine to the kidneys. It is the source of a person's power particularly when Taiji is used as a *martial* art. The middle *dan tian,* as mentioned above, is in the middle of the body in the area of the solar plexus and relates to general physical vitality. The upper *dan tian* is in the area of the pineal gland. To measure its precise position, draw an imaginary line from the tops of your ears through your head and another line from between the eyebrows (the *Third Eye Point*) straight to the back of your head. Where the two horizontal lines intersect is the location of the upper *dan tian*.

Before you begin

On the succeeding pages of this book there is a thorough description of seated Qigong and Taiji exercises intended for use by health care professionals, caregivers, and others who work with disabled, elderly, or post-surgical patients. It will take approximately 50 to 60 minutes to complete an entire set. This may be possible for you for your own wellness program but it will most likely not be possible when you are working with several individual patients each day. In that case, you might be able to use the sample lesson for beginners which combines exercises from Qigong and Taiji and should take no longer than 15 minutes to complete without rushing through them. Or, you may prefer to target each person's needs with one, two, or three exercises for each session.

Taiji and Qigong were designed to be practiced as any other daily habit such as brushing your teeth or combing your hair. Choose exercises for your patients that you think they will be able to learn easily and then encourage them to practice those exercises on their own. And, if at all possible, do these exercises *yourself* twice a day, once in the morning and once in the evening before you go to bed. You will accomplish more with regard to your overall physical, mental, and emotional health than you ever imagined possible. You will be an inspiration to your patients, and at night you'll sleep like a baby!

At the end of each of the exercise sections and after the acupressure points to be used with each set of exercises, you will notice that there is a graphic of a water pitcher.

This graphic is a reminder for you to stop for a minute and give your patients time to take a drink of water, even if they don't tell you they are thirsty. They may need rehydration because they have just stirred up toxins and will need to flush them out of their systems. For a more complete explanation of the role of water in relation to the exercises, please see the section in Chapter 4 entitled "Reducing fatigue and stress with water."

2

SEATED QIGONG QUICK PICKER-UPPERS

Exercises to Defeat Fatigue and Re-Energize

When it (qi) goes down it becomes quiet.
When it becomes quiet it will solidify.
When it becomes solidified it will begin to sprout.
After it has sprouted it will grow.
As it grows it will be pulled back again (to the upper regions).
When it has been pulled back it will reach the crown of the head.
Above, it will press against the crown of the head.
Above, it will press downwards.
Whoever follows this will live;
whoever acts contrary to it will die.

Translation of ancient inscription by Joseph Needham,
Science and Civilization in China (1983)

The history of Qigong

The term *Qigong* is made up of two characters, each with its own inherent meaning. Qigong is most often translated as "to work with qi" or "energy exercises." Each character that comprises the word, however, may embody other concepts depending on the context in which the character appears. The character for *qi* (*ch'i*) may also be used to mean steam, smoke, or breath. *Gong* (*kung*) may signify life energy, success, performance, or effect.

As with much of Chinese tradition and history, the exact origin of Qigong is not well documented, nor do Chinese scholars agree on the precise date or identification of the people involved in the development of this ancient healing art. We do know, however, that a form of Qigong was in use sometime during the Zhou Dynasty and the Warring States period because bamboo and bronze artifacts from that time refer to specific breathing practices. A silk scroll painted with figures of different genders and social classes performing dance-like postures similar to Qigong movements was excavated during an archaeological dig at a tomb in the Hunan Province of China. Inscriptions, though largely unreadable, appear to give instructions for each posture and the appropriate breathing technique associated with that movement.

Bodhidarma, who is generally considered to be the "father of martial arts," traveled from India to China where he taught the monks of the Shaolin Temple a series of Qigong type exercises combined with Buddhist meditative practices. These exercises have been preserved in the writings of the Shaolin monks and have led to the many legends regarding the superior fighting capabilities of these monks.

Hua Tuo, the most famous of all Chinese physicians (see Chapter 1) of the third century AD, designed a series of Qigong exercises for his patients called the "five animal forms." Hua Tuo created exercises based on the movements of deer, bears, monkeys, cranes, and tigers. He was confident that imitating the movements common to the deer would increase a person's gracefulness, mimicking the bear would ensure strength and balance, tiger exercises would enhance overall strength and quickness, crane movements would guarantee lightness of step and balance, and mirroring a monkey's activities would result in dexterity. Hua Tuo's belief in the role daily exercise plays in a person's overall health and fitness is well illustrated by the following quotations from this famous physician:

> *Flowing water never stagnates.*

> *A door hinge is never worm eaten.*

In other words, if one keeps moving energetically, that person's physical, mental, and spiritual functions will remain youthful and filled with *qi*. You will notice, however, when you begin the section on Qigong, that I have mixed Hua Tuo's deer, bear, and crane movements with other more recently developed exercises that I have found to be effective with my students. There are a number of wonderful books dealing with the original five animal forms, as well as newer adaptations of animal and combination exercises. Check with your local library or on the internet.

Sample lesson for beginners

The following is a sample collection of the exercises described in this book. I chose this particular combination because of the simplicity of the exercises. Each is presented in a way that will make it easy for you to explain the posture, movements, and benefits to your patient. You can read the instructions directly off the page if you wish since they are written as though directed toward an individual reading the book.

I have described the movements and given explanations of the benefits of each exercise so you won't have to flip back and forth during a session to find the information you need. By all means feel free to design a set of exercises that are the most appropriate for each of your patients. There is no need to begin with these exercises, but they are here to get you launched as you learn how to use seated Qigong and Taiji exercises in your work.

Qigong warm-up exercises

GATHERING QI

Benefits: This warm-up exercise brings the *qi* that may be trapped in other areas of the body into the lower *dan tian*. It is from this area that your patients will want to pull the energy up to their middle *dan tian* and, eventually, into the upper *dan tian,* the repository for mental and spiritual energy.

1. Sit comfortably with your back against the back of your chair, hips tucked slightly under. Make sure your legs are shoulder-width apart. Lift your head as though it is being pulled gently upward by a string attached to the ceiling.

2. Place your right hand over your lower *dan tian.* To be certain that your hand is in the right place, rest your right thumb on your navel. Your hand will then naturally rest on the lower *dan tian.* Place your left hand over your right.

3. Breathe in deeply through your nose and exhale through your mouth. Continue to breathe deeply but naturally for at least one full minute.

LIFTING YOUR QI

Benefits: By lifting each leg, the *qi* is being pushed upward into the trunk. As your patients place their feet back on the floor, the acupressure points on the soles of their feet are stimulated. See the diagram of foot acupressure points in Appendix B.

1. Keep your foot parallel to the floor as you lift it to the height of your abdomen or chest (Figure 2.1). Change feet and repeat.

2. Continue lifting your legs alternately for at least nine sets with each leg, if possible.

Note: The number of lifts can be increased as long as the thigh muscles don't become overly tense. Remember, like Taiji, Qigong should be performed in a relaxed way. Don't allow your patients to become tense as you lead them through the exercises.

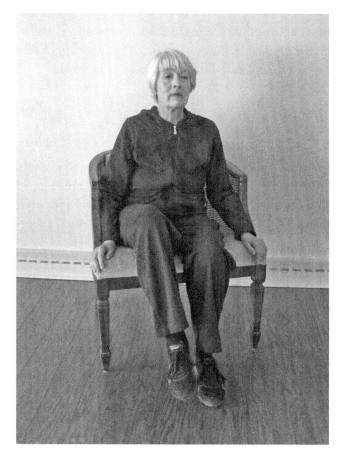

Figure 2.1 Lifting Your Qi

Centering Qi

Benefits: If *qi* has become trapped in an area of the body as the result of putting too much emphasis on one exercise or the other, or one side of the body or the other, this exercise will restore the *qi* to its proper balance. Breathing for this exercise is reverse breathing or pre-birth. Ask your patients to breathe in, contracting the diaphragm, then relaxing just the lower abdomen as stale air is released from their lungs.

1. Hold your hands palm up just above your lap, fingertips touching (Figure 2.2). Breathe in deeply through your nose while contracting your diaphragm. It is only in this one exercise that the diaphragm is *not* expanded during inhalations.

2. As you tighten your diaphragm and abdomen, raise your arms out to the side and up over your head to its center. Your palms are now facing the ceiling, fingers barely touching (Figure 2.3).

3. Allow your arms to descend gradually in an arc out to the side. As you do so, exhale until there is no breath left in your lungs and relax just the muscles of your lower abdomen.

4. Return your arms to the original position in front of the lowest part of your abdomen, palms upward.

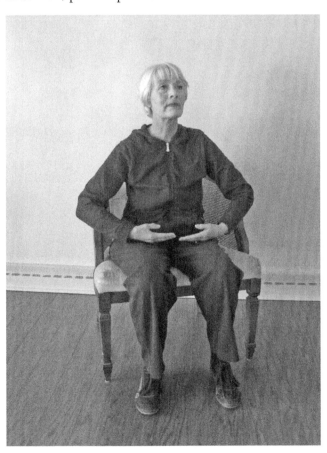

Figure 2.2 Centering Qi 1

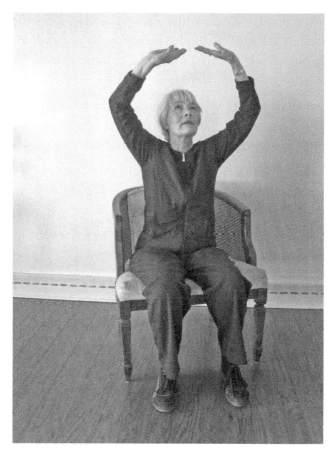

Figure 2.3 Centering Qi 2

Combined Qigong/Taiji exercises

HEAD, NECK, AND SHOULDERS

Benefits: Relaxes the muscles of the neck and realigns the cervical vertebrae.

Posture: Have your patients begin by sitting with their backs against the back of the chair. Legs should be shoulder-width apart, feet flat on the floor. Remind them to tuck their hips under slightly and curve their shoulders inward without hunching. Make sure they are holding their heads lightly on their necks as though their heads were suspended by a string from the ceiling.

Point of origin: Since you are targeting physical fatigue with these exercises, your patients must bring energy from the lower *dan tian* up and through the middle and upper *dan tians*. The neck is considered to be the link between the body and the mind. By concentrating on the movement of the *qi* as it moves through the center of the body, it will be possible for your patients to ease the tension between their minds and bodies that may be causing stiffness and pain in shoulder and neck muscles.

Visualization for your patients: Imagine that your neck muscles are as supple as an infant's and that your head is a light ball perched on a flexible stalk.

Warning: I have had patients who expressed some discomfort when performing this exercise but who had neither an injury nor surgery in the neck area, so please use caution when introducing this exercise.

1. Breathe in while your head is upright.

2. Lower your head gently to your chest while breathing out.

3. Return your head to the center, breathe in again, and lower your head gently backwards as you breathe out. Repeat nine times, counting the forward and backward motion as one.

4. Now, let your head drop down toward your right shoulder. Return your head to the center and then relax your neck muscles as you lower your head to your left shoulder.

5. You will finish with your head tilted to the right. Circle your head down to your chest and then back to the left. Do not lean your head backwards while circling.

6. Continue circling your head right to left for a total of nine times.

7. Lean your head over your left shoulder, then to your right, and so on for a total of nine times.

8. Again, beginning on the left side, circle your head from left to chest to the right shoulder for a total of nine times.

9. Look over your right shoulder and turn your eyes in the same direction as though you were trying to look at someone standing behind you. Now, glance over your left shoulder. Continue alternating side to side nine times.

10. Look over your left shoulder and tilt your head so that you are looking up into the corner where the wall and ceiling meet. Repeat the same movement to the right and continue alternating for a total of nine times.

11. Raise your shoulders toward your ears. Allow them to drop abruptly. This is a particularly good exercise for stiff shoulders. If, however, you experience pain when dropping your shoulders, lower them gently instead. Repeat the shoulder lifts and drops nine times.

FLOWER BUD OPENS

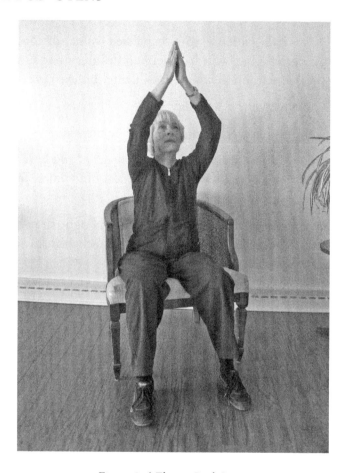

Figure 2.4 Flower Bud Opens

Benefits: While lifting the rib cage, the chest is opened to the fullest extent, allowing for a deeper inhalation.

Posture: Direct your patients to begin in the original posture. As the arms are brought above the head and swung to the back, make sure your patients arch away from their chairs.

Point of origin: The point of origin is the upper *dan tian*. Direct your patients to imagine that the *shen* (refer to section on the *Three Treasures* in Chapter 1 for an explanation of *shen*) is like a ball spinning rapidly, throwing off sparks of energy throughout their heads, upper chests, necks, and shoulders.

Visualization for your patients: Think about the first yawn of the morning. Your chest opens wide as clean, clear air enters your lungs.

1. Begin with your hands in a prayer position (that is, palms pressed together, fingers pointed straight upwards) in front of your solar plexus.

2. Raise your hands above your head, keeping your palms pressed together (Figure 2.4).

3. When your elbows are straight, open your arms to the side, sweeping them in an arc to the furthest point possible behind you. As your arms being to circle out to the side, arch your back away from the back of the chair.

4. Return your arms to the prayer position and repeat nine times.

Golden Cockerel

Benefits: Repetition of this movement trims and tones the leg muscles, particularly those of the thigh. Since it is the abdominal muscles that are used in the leg lifts, the abdomen itself is also firmed and the belly tightened.

Posture: Direct your patients to sit in the same position as in the previous exercise.

Point of origin: Instruct your patients to use the energy from the lower *dan tian* and direct it downward through their working leg.

Visualization for your patients: Imagine the *qi* flowing along the meridian on the outside of your leg as you lift. The *qi* then returns up the inside of your thigh as you return your foot to the floor.

1. Begin with your right leg. Breathe in, lift your rib cage, and tighten your diaphragm and abdomen. Concentrate on the action of the muscles of your abdomen and the muscles on the top of your thigh as you bend your knee and lift your leg to the level of your abdomen or chest. By tightening these sets of muscles, your thigh is pulled upward toward your torso.

2. Hold your working leg in position for the duration of the inward breath and then lower your leg slowly as you release your breath and relax your diaphragm. Always lower your leg more slowly than you

lifted it. This will increase the tension on the thigh muscles, trimming and toning your thighs more quickly.

3. Now, change to your left leg. Repeat the breath in, the lift of your rib cage, and the contraction of your diaphragm and abdomen as you raise your leg toward your chest. Remember to lower your leg more slowly than you lifted it and in time with the exhalation of your breath and relaxation of your abdominal muscles.

4. Continue alternating the lifts until you have completed nine lifts with each leg for a total of 18 lifts.

BRUSHING TREE TRUNK

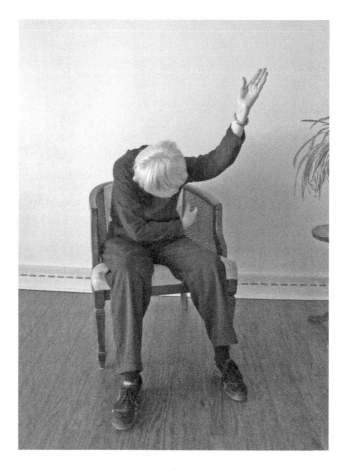

Figure 2.5 Brushing Tree Trunk

Benefits: Balances the right and left hemispheres of the brain, thereby ridding the mind of distractions and uncertainty.

Posture: Direct your patients to begin in the same position as in the previous exercise.

Point of origin: This exercise will stimulate the movement of *qi* from the upper *dan tian* which is located in the upper center of the head.

Visualization for your patients: Think about the *qi* as it circulates evenly in and around the right and left hemispheres of the brain, balancing and energizing both creativity and rational thought.

1. Begin by raising your arms until your elbows are straight.

2. Leave your left arm extended while you swing your right arm downward as you bend from the waist, then swing your right arm across your body until your elbow is bent and your arm brushes your thighs (Figure 2.5).

3. Turn your head so that you are looking up and over your right shoulder.

4. Return your right arm to its upward extension and swing your left arm down across your body while bending over from the waist. Look up and over your left shoulder.

5. Repeat nine times on each side for a total of 18 brushes.

CENTERING QI

Benefits: This exercise centers the energy and rebalances the body.

Posture: Direct your patients to sit as in the previous exercise.

Point of origin: While engaging in continuous deep diaphragmatic breathing, the energy or *qi* from the lower *dan tian* is being pulled up through the middle *dan tian* and, finally, all the way to the upper *dan tian* that contains mental energy.

Visualization for your patients: Imagine that you are collecting the *qi* and bits of energy from all over your body, returning them to a "neutral" position at the lower *dan tian* so that none will be lost or trapped elsewhere in the body.

1. Hold your hands palm up just above your lap, fingertips touching (see Figure 2.2, page 27). Breathe in deeply through your nose while contracting your diaphragm. It is only in this one exercise that the diaphragm is *not* expanded during inhalations.

2. As you tighten your diaphragm and abdomen, raise your arms out to the side and up over your head to its center. Your palms are now facing the ceiling, fingers barely touching (see Figure 2.3, page 28).

3. Allow your arms to descend gradually in an arc out to the side. As you do so, exhale until there is no breath left in your lungs and relax just the muscles of your lower abdomen.

4. Return your arms to the original position in front of the lowest part of your abdomen, palms upward.

Acupressure points

Triple Warmer Meridian No. 15—Heavenly Rejuvenation

This pressure point is midway between the base of the neck and the outside edge of the shoulder at approximately one half inch (1.25cm) to the back of the shoulder muscle. Direct your patients to press firmly on this spot with the middle finger of the opposite hand for at least 30 seconds while breathing deeply in and out.

Benefits: Much of our stress is experienced as tension in the shoulders and stiffness in the neck, so this point may be used whenever there is pain or stiffness in these areas.

Conception Vessel Meridian No. 17—Sea of Tranquility

Help your patients locate this acupressure point by asking them to measure three thumb-widths up from the base of their breastbones along its center. Make sure your patients press firmly for a full minute. They may repeat the use of this point as often as necessary.

Benefits: If a person is prone to panic attacks, this point should be used at the onset of the attack. This pressure point is also useful to relieve hiccups, nervousness, and general anxiety. Direct your patients to sit in a comfortable chair, breathe deeply, and concentrate on each breath until they begin to feel calm.

Governing Vessel Meridian No. 20—One Hundred Meeting Point

Governing Vessel Meridian No. 19—Posterior Summit

Governing Vessel Meridian No. 21—Anterior Summit

All three of these points are on the top of the head and are the most effective antidepressant acupressure points on the body. Help your patients locate *One Hundred Meeting Point*, by running their fingers to the top of their heads from behind each ear until they find a sizeable indentation. There is another hollow approximately one inch (2.5cm) to the front of the *One Hundred Meeting Point* and another about the same distance to the back of the *One Hundred Meeting Point*. The front point is the *Anterior Summit* and the furthest to the back of the head is the *Posterior Summit*. Suggest that your patients press firmly for a full minute on one or all of these points. They may use these acupressure points often.

Benefits: If the patients you are working with are having memory problems or suffer from depression, stress-induced headaches, or vertigo, you will want to suggest that they utilize these three points frequently and consistently. Remember to suggest that they combine the use of these points with deep diaphragmatic breathing while sitting comfortably in a quiet area.

MEDITATIVE RELAXATION

Benefits: The following mental exercises will relax the body, clear the mind, and restore the spirit to a state of balance and calm.

Posture: Remind your patients to check their postures. Make sure their backs are against the back of the chair, feet are flat on the floor, toes turned slightly inward, and their legs are shoulder-width apart. Make certain that they are sitting up straight so that their heads are lightly suspended on their necks and their shoulders are rounded slightly forward but not hunched.

Point of origin: Encourage your patients to concentrate on bringing the *qi* or energy upward from their lower *dan tian*. They will be moving their energy with their minds through the middle *dan tian* that regulates the emotions and then to the upper *dan tian* that controls the mind and spirit.

Visualization for your patients: Imagine yourself floating on a cloud. Soothing, revitalizing energy passes from the top of your head, through your arms and trunk, and, finally, into your legs from where the *qi* flows back into the earth.

1. Close your eyes. Take a deep breath, expanding your diaphragm. Picture a flow of energy traveling up to the top of your head. Now, allow the energy to stream downward flooding your head, neck, and face. Breathe out, gently contracting your diaphragm. Take two more deep, gentle breaths as you continue to visualize the energy flowing in and around your head and neck.

2. Now, mentally push the energy from your neck down into your shoulders, arms, and hands while you breathe deeply in and out for a total of three cleansing breaths.

3. Take the energy from the shoulders and push it into your trunk, allowing the healing energy to circle in and around your organs and to travel up and down your spine. Take three long breaths while you envision the movement of the *qi*.

4. Direct the flow of energy from your trunk down into your hips, thighs, and knees. Allow the energy to circulate, soothing and relaxing overworked muscles and joints. Time the flow of the energy by taking three deep breaths in and out using the post-birth method. Remember that the "post-birth" method means your diaphragm is expanded while breathing in, and contracted when you are breathing out.

5. Then, direct the *qi* that you have released with your thoughts and, breathing deeply, send it into the lowest part of your legs, the calves, ankles, and, finally, the feet.

Note: We all exchange energy with our environment without realizing that the exchange is happening. Electromagnetic energy rises from the earth and is absorbed into the body through the soles of the feet. The energy or *qi* coursing through our bodies is returned to the earth as it moves through our upper bodies, down our legs, and out through the soles of our feet.

Introduction to Qigong exercise

If you are familiar with Taiji, you will notice as you go through the following section of exercises that many of the individual movements resemble those used in Taiji exercises. We can only speculate about the reason for these similarities. We do know that Hua Tuo had published his book of internal medicine with a description of his healing exercises by the third century AD. Historians tell us that Zhang Sanfeng did not design his martial art form, Taijiquan, until at least the 13th century AD. It is likely that Zhang Sanfeng was familiar with the writings of China's most eminent physician, so it is perhaps not surprising that he incorporated some of the doctor's Qigong exercises into his martial art form.

The difference between the two systems, of course, is that Taijiquan was never intended for anything except martial applications. Qigong, on the other hand, was the creation of a practicing physician whose only interest was to improve the health of his patients. Some of the exercises in this section were devised specifically for certain organs of the body; others are intended to increase the flow of *qi* or to tone and strengthen muscles and joints.

Each of the sections begins with the same warm-up exercises. It is important to help your patients understand that they should release the *qi* and send this energy throughout their trunks and limbs so that all the succeeding exercises will have the desired effect.

The exercise *Gathering Qi* is the first and most basic of the Qigong warm-up exercises. Note the position of the hands at the area of the navel. Each new human being forms around one central area of the mother's womb. It is here that the fetus is attached to its mother, receiving nourishment and growing cell by cell throughout the pregnancy. That attachment point, of course, is the umbilical cord, remaining in adults at the navel. That is why the Chinese spend so much time and effort on stimulating the *qi* that resides just below the belly button. This area of the body remains the primary reservoir of *qi*, just as it was before birth.

After your patients "gather the *qi*"— in other words wake up their energy—you and they will use the exercise *Stimulating Qi* to bring the energy up through the trunk and out to the arms, all the way to the fingertips. The gentle slaps used in *Spreading Qi* encourage not only the spread of energy but also increased circulation to outer areas. *Lifting Your Qi* continues to push energy up through the trunk and stimulates acupressure points along the soles of the feet (see Appendix B). As with all the other series of exercises, each section ends with *Centering Qi* to ensure the return of energy to the lower *dan tian*.

There are three exercises that specifically target the kidneys. Kidneys are two fist-sized organs that are located just above the waist. Kidneys function as filters for the body, removing waste and excess fluid. These kidney-specific exercises are *Touching Toes, Bending Backward, Wash the Marrow with One Hand* and *Shooting the Bow*. The bending and arching of the lower back in *Touching Toes, Bending Backward* stimulates kidney function while stretching hamstrings and calves.

Wash the Marrow with One Hand is believed to be beneficial for the kidneys in their filtering activities and for the adrenals. Adrenals act as the body's reserve tank. Energy held in reserve when not needed can be released and distributed throughout the body when physical, mental, emotional, or chemical stress is placed on the body. Obviously, then, this exercise is one that you can recommend when your patients express feelings of fatigue, or they may use it on a daily basis to ensure the proper dissemination of *qi* as they deal with day-to-day stressors.

Shooting the Bow is the third exercise in this Qigong section that is particularly useful in maintaining the proper functioning of the kidneys. This exercise also benefits all the meridians of the body and stimulates the normal activity of internal organs. *Shooting the Bow* works the muscles in the arms and shoulders, tightening those areas of the arms that tend to become flabby as we age.

The exercise *Balancing the Triple Warmer* is a multi-purpose exercise that is beneficial for an astounding number of organs. "Triple" refers to the basic function of this exercise as it targets the stomach, lungs, and heart. But, in addition to those three organs, *Balancing the Triple Warmer* also benefits the spleen and the liver.

The spleen is the most important organ in terms of our resistance to disease. It is the largest lymph organ in the body. Blood passing through the spleen comes into contact with lymphocytes whose main job is to attack foreign invaders such as harmful bacteria and viruses. For those born with a dysfunctional spleen or who have had spleens removed through surgery, exposure to contaminants in the air is a serious situation. A person without a spleen is missing his/her most important organ in the fight against disease.

The liver is no less important to the proper functioning of the body. The Hepatitis Information Network (www.hepnet.com) lists the following functions of the liver:

- regulation, synthesis, and secretion of many of the substances important in maintaining the body's normal, healthy state

- storage of important nutrients, vitamins, and minerals

- purification, transformation, and clearance of drugs, toxins, and waste products.

The exercise *Punching with a Steady Gaze* is beneficial for the functioning of the liver, destroying toxins and allowing faster healing after illness or injury. For additional protection and stimulation of the spleen, use the exercise *Raising Each Arm* often for your patients, along with *Balancing the Triple Warmer*.

You may use any of the Qigong exercises for yourself or your patients in any combination you choose. They are grouped, however, by difficulty, so that the level one exercises are those that I have found to be the easiest to master, with level two and level three of progressive complexity. Once you have given a sufficient amount of time to learning each of the exercises, you will be able to combine them in a daily routine that is most beneficial for your patients (for you too, of course!) and that targets their particular needs. Remember always to begin each session with the warm-up exercises. Move through the exercises slowly, calmly and with concentration, directing your patients to do the same. They will benefit not only in the level of their physical fitness and resistance to disease but I am confident that you and your patients will also experience improved concentration, mental acuity, stability of your emotions, and a greater spiritual awareness.

Note: Remind your patients to replenish their fluids often during the exercise sessions if their medical conditions permit.

Level one Qigong exercises

I have included all the warm-up exercises from the previous section for your convenience. Each of the following Qigong exercise levels includes these exercises so you won't have to flip back to the opening section.

Always begin the exercise session with your patients with all or some of the warm-ups. If time is an issue, use two or three of the following exercises that you feel will give them the best warming. I encourage you to experiment until you find the right combination for those instances when time is limited. Remember, you can read the instructions directly off the page if you wish since they are written as though directed toward an individual reading the book.

Qigong warm-up exercises

GATHERING QI

Benefits: This warm-up exercise brings the *qi* that may be trapped in other areas of the body into the lower *dan tian*. It is from this area that the energy should be pulled upward to the middle *dan tian* and, eventually, into the upper *dan tian,* the repository for mental and spiritual energy.

1. Sit comfortably with your back against the back of your chair, hips tucked slightly under. Make sure your legs are shoulder-width apart. Lift your head as though it is being pulled gently upward by a string attached to the ceiling.

2. Place your right hand over your lower *dan tian.* To be certain that your hand is in the right place, rest your right thumb on your navel. Your hand will then naturally rest on the lower *dan tian.* Place your left hand over your right.

3. Breathe in deeply through your nose and exhale through your mouth. Continue to breathe deeply but naturally for at least one full minute.

STIMULATING QI

Benefits: As your patients' arms are swung back and forth, the *qi* from the lower *dan tian* will surge upwards and out to their fingertips. The forward swing lifts the energy to the middle *dan tian* and then out along the arms. This exercise is both soothing and energizing.

1. Check your posture to be sure your feet are still shoulder-width apart and your hips are tucked under so that the small of your back is resting against the back of your chair.

2. Make certain that your arms are on the outside of the arms of your chair at a sufficient distance so you don't bang against the sides as you swing your arms.

3. Begin by swinging your arms backward. Allow both arms to swing forward naturally. Don't try to time your breathing with this exercise. Continue to breathe in through your nose and expel the toxins out through your mouth in your normal breathing rhythm.

4. Begin with at least 36 swings. You may increase the number of swings as you progress.

SPREADING QI

Benefits: This exercise will seem familiar because it is something we all do unconsciously and automatically when we're cold. By gently slapping their thighs and arms, your patients will be increasing the circulation in their limbs and distributing the *qi* throughout their bodies.

1. Begin by crossing your arms. Slap your arms gently from the elbows up to the shoulders and back down to the elbows again. Do not try to time your breathing to the slaps.

2. Sit forward on your chair so that you won't hit your arms while you do this exercise. Swing your arms out to the sides and then slap them against your thighs. Continue to breathe naturally—not in time with your arm movements.

3. Start with 36 slaps on your arms and 36 on your legs.

Note: Your patients may increase the pressure of their slaps or build up to a larger number if you judge it is safe to do so, but never to the point of soreness or bruising.

LIFTING YOUR QI

Benefits: By lifting each leg, your patients are pushing the *qi* upward into their trunks. As the feet are placed back on the floor, the acupressure points on the soles of the feet are stimulated. See the diagram of foot acupressure points in Appendix B.

1. Sit back against the back of your chair again. Tuck your hips underneath you so that the small of your back is supported against the back of your chair. Feet and legs should be shoulder-width apart.

2. Keep your foot parallel to the floor as you lift it to the height of your abdomen or chest (see Figure 2.1, page 26). Change feet and repeat.

3. Continue lifting your legs alternately for at least nine sets with each leg, if possible.

4. Again, you may increase the number of lifts as long as your thigh muscles don't become overly tense. Qigong should be performed in a relaxed way; don't allow yourself to become tense as you go through the exercises.

Centering Qi

Benefits: If the *qi* has become trapped in an area of the body as a result of putting too much emphasis on one exercise or the other or on one side of the body or the other, this exercise will restore the *qi* to its proper balance. Remember, breathing for this exercise is reverse breathing or pre-birth. When your patients breathe in, remind them to contract the diaphragm, then relax just the lower abdomen when the stale air is released from their lungs out through the mouth.

1. Hold your hands palm up just above your lap, fingertips touching (see Figure 2.2, page 27). Breathe in deeply through your nose while contracting your diaphragm. It is only in this one exercise that the diaphragm is *not* expanded during inhalations.

2. As you tighten your diaphragm and abdomen, raise your arms out to the side and up over your head to its center. Your palms are now facing the ceiling, fingers barely touching (see Figure 2.3, page 28).

3. Allow your arms to descend gradually in an arc out to the side. As you do so, exhale until there is no breath left in your lungs and relax just the muscles of your lower abdomen.

4. Return your arms to the original position in front of the lowest part of your abdomen, palms upward.

Qigong exercises

The Crane

Benefits: This exercise is part of a standard Qigong meditation. Your patients should be as relaxed and attentive to the movement of their breath as possible. Encourage your patients to concentrate and to avoid letting their minds wander into worrisome thoughts. If you have eliminated all environmental distractions before you begin this session with your patients and if this "experiencing" meditation is practiced consistently by your patients on their own in between their meetings with you, they will achieve an improved state of tranquility.

1. As you breathe in through your nose, expand your diaphragm. Imagine that your hands are gathering the cleansing *qi* into your lower *dan tian*.

2. As you breathe in, gently press your back into the chair.

3. As you blow out the toxins, imagine that your hands are helping to push the breath out through your mouth. Move forward and downward so that your back is no longer pressed against the back of your chair. In other words, rock slightly forward and lean ever so slightly toward your thighs.

4. Repeat for at least a full minute. If you can manage it, increase the time to five minutes.

THE TURTLE

Benefits: These meditative exercises all contribute to reducing stress and fatigue. Because they are so gentle and performed so slowly, internal organs are nourished and the stress placed on these organs as the result of lifestyle, injury, illness, or surgery will be greatly lessened.

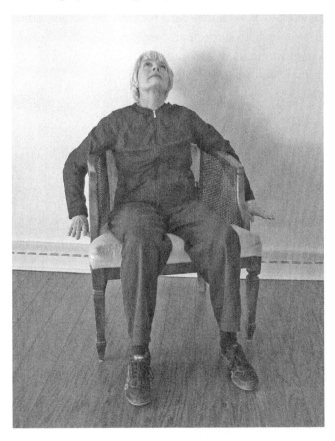

Figure 2.6 The Turtle

1. Continue the gentle swaying, rocking movement that you used in the previous exercise. Shorten your neck as you breathe a cleansing breath into your lower abdomen.

2. Your back should remain pressed against the back of your chair during the inward breath. Feel the breath with your hands (still pressed against your lower abdomen) as the cleansing breath enters through your nose.

3. As you breathe out, pull slightly away from the chair and stretch your neck upward (Figure 2.6).

4. Continue the movements for at least a full minute, extending to five minutes when you have the time and feel that you have perfected the neck retractions as well as the swaying/rocking motion.

THE DEER

Benefits: This exercise will benefit your patients in two ways. Deep breathing will flood the system with oxygen and enhance the movement of the *qi*. In addition, these movements will stimulate the energy from the lower *dan tian* (the *jing*), for increased sexual or physical energy.

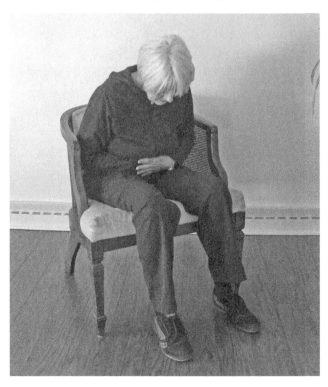

Figure 2.7 The Deer

1. Remain in the usual posture with your feet flat on the floor, the small of your back pressed against the back of your chair. Keep your hands on your lower abdomen to simulate the drawing of energy into your abdomen.

2. Lift upward with the muscles around your tailbone as you inhale and expand your abdomen. As you blow the air out of your mouth, tighten your abdominal muscles and lean forward slightly with a gentle rocking motion (Figure 2.7).

3. Repeat the motions, the breathing, and the muscle contractions for at least a full minute. If time allows, work up to five minutes.

BALANCING THE TRIPLE WARMER

Benefits: Three organs comprise the "Triple Warmer" or "Triple Burner"—the heart, the lungs, and the stomach. This exercise, however, goes beyond these three organs to stimulate and regulate the spleen and the liver as well.

1. Begin in the same posture as in the exercise above.

2. Lace your fingers, lifting your arms upward over your head. At the same time, roll up on the balls of your feet.

3. Press your heels back onto the floor as you bring your hands to the top of your head.

4. Stretch your arms over your head, twisting your hands so the palms are facing toward the ceiling. At the same time, roll up onto the balls of your feet.

5. Continue rolling up on the balls of your feet, pressing your laced hands (palms up) toward the ceiling, alternating with palms down, pressing gently on the top of the head and lowering your heels to the floor.

SHOOTING THE BOW

Benefits: Once again, your patients will be stimulating meridians and internal organs during this exercise. Their arm and shoulder muscles will be stretched and tightened, helping to eliminate underarm flabbiness. This is also an excellent exercise for improving breathing and strengthening lungs. Some Chinese medical practitioners believe that this exercise also benefits the kidneys.

1. Check that you haven't moved away from the back of your chair; reposition your feet and your back if necessary.

2. Bring your hands under your chin with backs facing (Figure 2.8). Push out with your right arm to the right side and turn your head so that you are looking toward your extended arm.

3. Open your right hand so that your index finger is pointed to the side while the middle finger, ring finger, and little finger are curled slightly toward your palm.

4. At the same time your right arm is moving out to the right, close your left hand into a fist and press your left elbow out to the side so that both arms are parallel to the floor (Figure 2.9).

5. Reverse and repeat at least nine times on each side.

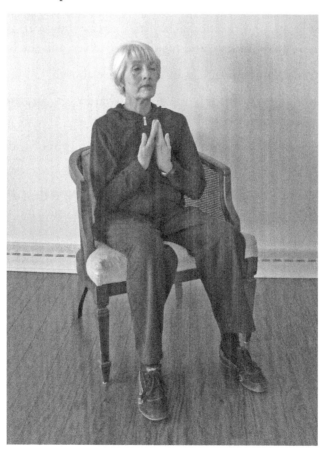

Figure 2.8 Shooting the Bow 1

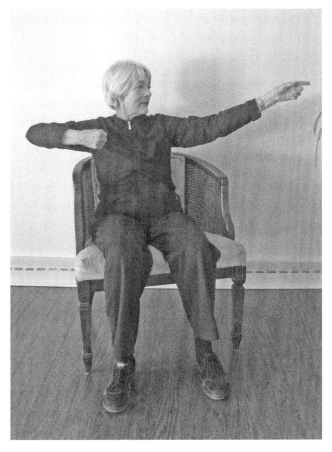

Figure 2.9 Shooting the Bow 2

Big Bear Turns from Side to Side

Benefits: *Big Bear Turns from Side to Side* helps to regulate heart rate and exercises the lungs. This exercise is also beneficial in trimming the waist. Hips and abdominal and lower back muscles will be tightened and stretched. If your patients are experiencing back pain or stiffness, this exercise—performed gently, of course—will be of great benefit in releasing those overly tight muscles.

1. Plant your feet firmly on the floor, shoulder-width apart, and press the small of your back against the back of your chair by tucking your hips underneath you. Take a deep breath through your nose before you move to the next step.

2. Blow out through your nose as you bend forward from your hips and swing your torso to the left. At the same time, turn your head so that you are looking at the wall to your left.

3. Swing back to the middle, shifting your eyes to the wall directly in front of you, and breathe in through your nose. Do not raise your back but, rather, swing directly to the right in the same bent-over position. Remember to turn your head in the direction of the movement so that this time you are looking at the wall to your right.

4. Lift up and return to your original upright position. Again, take a deep breath in through your nose and swing your torso over your right thigh as you exhale and look toward the wall to your right. Swing to the left and then return to your upright position.

5. Repeat this gentle pendulum motion, alternating sides for a minimum of 12 repetitions. It is most important that you swing to the left and to the right an equal number of times.

Note: If your patients experience any serious discomfort or pain, stop immediately and have them take several deep breaths before continuing the exercise session. Reduce or increase the number of swings depending upon your patients' physical condition and on how they tell you they feel when they finish this exercise. You and your patients should set the pace based on what you observe and what they tell you after a few repetitions.

TOUCHING TOES, BENDING BACKWARD

Benefits: This exercise will stretch the back muscles, drawing the *qi* into the entire upper body. The bending and arching movements stimulate the kidneys and stretch the hamstrings and calves. Because your patients are seated for these movements, some adaptation of the original is necessary. I leave it to you to determine exactly how to modify this exercise based on the physical condition of each of your patients.

1. Check your posture again to be sure you haven't moved out of position.

2. Begin by inhaling deeply in through your nose (as you bend forward, start exhaling so that you will have blown out all your breath before you return to your starting position).

3. Rounding your back slightly, bend forward over your thighs, sliding your hands down the outside of your legs until you touch your toes. At the same time, pull your toes back so that you are resting on your

heels. Pulling your toes back will stretch and lengthen the muscles in your calves.

4. Return to the upright position, keeping your back slightly rounded so that you move upward vertebra by vertebra and breathe in as you are doing so.

5. Once your back is straight, arch away from the back of the chair. Lean back as far as possible, allowing your head to tip backwards at the same time and breathe out.

Note: If your patients have had a neck injury or back or neck surgery, be cautious in introducing them to this particular exercise.

CENTERING QI

Benefits: If the *qi* has become trapped in an area of the body as a result of putting too much emphasis on one exercise or the other, or one side of the body or the other, this exercise will restore the *qi* to its proper balance. Remind your patients that the proper breathing for this exercise is reverse breathing or pre-birth. They should be contracting their diaphragms when breathing in and then relaxing just the lower abdomen when they release the stale air from their lungs.

1. Hold your hands palm up just above your lap, fingertips touching (see Figure 2.2, page 27). Breathe in deeply through your nose while contracting your diaphragm. It is only in this one exercise that the diaphragm is *not* expanded during inhalations.

2. As you tighten your diaphragm and abdomen, raise your arms out to the side and up over your head to its center. Your palms are now facing the ceiling, fingers barely touching (see Figure 2.3, page 28).

3. Allow your arms to descend gradually in an arc out to the side. As you do so, exhale until there is no breath left in your lungs and relax just the muscles of your lower abdomen.

4. Return your arms to the original position in front of the lowest part of your abdomen, palms upward.

Level two Qigong exercises

Before you and your patients begin the Qigong exercises, remember always to use at least one or two of the following warm-ups if you don't have time for all four of them. Include *Centering Qi* at the end whatever else you may have to skip, or if you have to reduce the number of repetitions. The rest of the exercise session will benefit your patients greatly if you consistently teach these exercises in the proper order. Patients may become confused if you change the order before they feel comfortable with the exercises.

Qigong warm-up exercises

Before you begin the Qigong exercises, introduce at least one or two of the following warm-ups when the session isn't long enough for all four of them. Remember to include *Centering Qi* at the end.

GATHERING QI

Benefits: This warm-up exercise brings the *qi* that may be trapped in other areas of the body into the lower *dan tian*. It is from this area that the energy should be pulled upward to the middle *dan tian* and, eventually, into the upper *dan tian,* the repository for mental and spiritual energy.

1. Sit comfortably with your back against the back of your chair, hips tucked slightly under. Make sure your legs are shoulder-width apart. Lift your head as though it is being pulled gently upward by a string attached to the ceiling.

2. Place your right hand over your lower *dan tian.* To be certain that your hand is in the right place, rest your right thumb on your navel. Your hand will then naturally rest on the lower *dan tian.* Place your left hand over your right.

3. Breathe in deeply through your nose and exhale through your mouth. Continue to breathe deeply but naturally for at least one full minute.

STIMULATING QI

Benefits: As your patients swing their arms back and forth, the *qi* from the lower *dan tian* will surge upwards and out to their fingertips. The forward swing lifts the energy to the middle *dan tian* and then out along their arms. This exercise is both soothing and energizing.

4. Check your posture to be sure your feet are still shoulder-width apart and your hips are tucked under so that the small of your back is resting against the back of your chair.

5. Make certain that your arms are on the outside of the arms of your chair at a sufficient distance so you don't bang against the sides as you swing your arms.

6. Begin by swinging your arms backward. Allow both arms to swing forward naturally. Don't try to time your breathing with this exercise. Continue to breathe in through your nose and expel the toxins out through your mouth in your normal breathing rhythm.

7. Begin with at least 36 swings. You may increase the number of swings as you progress.

SPREADING QI

Benefits: This exercise will seem familiar to your patients because it is something all of us unconsciously and automatically do when we're cold. By gently slapping their thighs and arms, your patients' circulation will increase in their limbs and distribute the *qi* throughout their bodies.

1. Begin by crossing your arms. Slap your arms gently from the elbows up to the shoulders and back down to the elbows again. Do not try to time your breathing to the slaps.

2. Sit forward on your chair so that you won't hit your arms while you do this exercise. Swing your arms out to the sides and then slap them against your thighs. Continue to breathe naturally—not in time with your arm movements. You may increase the pressure of your slaps but never to the point of soreness or bruising.

3. Start with 36 slaps on your arms and 36 on your legs.

Note: You may suggest to your patients to increase the pressure of the slaps, or direct them to build up to a larger number but never to the point of soreness or bruising.

LIFTING YOUR QI

Benefits: By lifting each leg, your patients are moving their *qi* upward into their trunks. As each foot returns to the floor, the acupressure points on the soles of the feet are stimulated. See the diagram of foot acupressure points in Appendix B.

1. Sit back against the back of your chair again. Tuck your hips underneath you so that the small of your back is supported against the back of your chair. Feet and legs should be shoulder-width apart.

2. Keep your foot parallel to the floor as you lift it to the height of your abdomen or chest. Change feet and repeat.

3. Continue lifting your legs alternately for at least nine sets with each leg, if possible.

4. Again, you may increase the number of lifts as long as your thigh muscles don't become overly tense. Remember, like Taiji, Qigong should be performed in a relaxed way. Don't allow yourself to become tense as you go through the exercises.

Centering Qi

Benefits: If the *qi* has become trapped in an area of the body as a result of putting too much emphasis on one exercise or the other, or one side of the body or the other, this exercise will restore the *qi* to its proper balance. Remind your patients that, for this exercise, they should use reverse or pre-birth breathing. When they breathe in, they should tighten their diaphragms and then relax just the lower abdomen when they breathe out, releasing stale air from their lungs.

1. Hold your hands palm up just above your lap, fingertips touching (see Figure 2.2, page 27). Breathe in deeply through your nose while contracting your diaphragm. It is only in this one exercise that the diaphragm is *not* expanded during inhalations.

2. As you tighten your diaphragm and abdomen, raise your arms out to the side and up over your head to its center. Your palms are now facing the ceiling, fingers barely touching (see Figure 2.3, page 28).

3. Allow your arms to descend gradually in an arc out to the side. As you do so, exhale until there is no breath left in your lungs and relax just the muscles of your lower abdomen.

4. Return your arms to the original position in front of the lowest part of your abdomen, palms upward.

Qigong exercises

RAISING EACH ARM

Benefits: This exercise is said to be particularly helpful in regulating the spleen. In addition, your patients will strengthen and stretch their shoulder and arm muscles. Repeated daily, these movements will trim their upper arms and release any shoulder tension they may be experiencing.

1. Check your posture. Remember your hips should be tucked under slightly so that the small of your back is against the back of your chair. Feet should be shoulder-width apart, head and neck stretched upward.

2. Begin with your right hand, palm facing the ceiling, resting on the crown of your head. The left arm, palm facing downward and elbow bent, should be held alongside the left rib cage.

3. Press upward with your right hand as you push downward with your left.

4. Keep your eyes straight forward, breathing in deeply through your nose and expanding your diaphragm as you stretch your arms in opposite directions. Breathe out through your mouth as you bring both arms back to the beginning position.

5. Continue for a total of 18 repetitions unless you are experiencing discomfort. Patients should talk with their physician before using this exercise if they have suffered a serious neck or shoulder injury or if they have had surgery in this general area.

WASHING THE MARROW WITH ONE HAND

Benefits: This exercise is beneficial for the proper functioning of the adrenals and the kidneys. The purpose of the arm movements in *Washing the Marrow with One Hand* is to balance the *yin* and the *yang*. The active arm begins at the *bai hui*, which is the acupressure point known as the *One Hundred Meeting Point*. This is the point on the body where multiple energy points converge so that connecting at this point makes it possible to move the *qi* easily up and down the body.

1. Always check your posture before beginning each exercise. In this case, however, you will need to move away from the back of your chair.

2. Breathe in deeply as you slowly move your left arm around your back until your left hand is resting against the small of your back.

3. At the same time, lift your right arm over your head until your right hand is about six inches (15cm) above your head (Figure 2.10).

4. Begin exhaling as you move your right hand slowly and with great concentration from the top of your head, down the center of your body, and out over your lap.

5. Draw your right arm back toward your abdomen while bringing your left arm to the front. Rest both hands on your thighs, take a couple of deep, slow breaths, and relax for a moment.

6. Now, take a deep breath and bring your right arm behind you slowly and gently until the back of your right hand is resting on the small of your back. Bring your left arm above your head so that your hand, palm down, is about six inches (15cm) above the crown. Bring your left hand slowly down the front of your body and out over your lap.

7. Return both hands to your thighs and rest again for a moment.

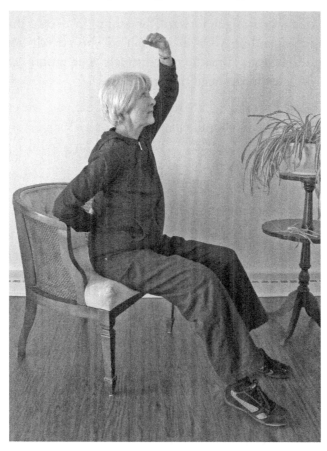

Figure 2.10 Washing the Marrow with One Hand

WISE OWL GAZES BACKWARD

Benefits: This is a very effective exercise for reducing stress and curing fatigue. This exercise is especially soothing for neck and shoulder tension. It is similar to the head and neck exercises in the Taiji relaxation section, but because this is a brief version of the other exercise, it can be performed in a shorter period of time and with greater concentration.

1. Again, check your posture. Rest your hands on the top of your thighs and take a deep, cleansing breath.

2. Turn your head as far to the right as possible while taking a breath in through your nose and expanding your diaphragm. At the same time, look over your shoulder at the wall behind you.

3. Return your head to the center while blowing out the toxins. Stop for a moment and focus on the wall directly in front of you.

4. Now, turn your head to the left, inhaling, and look over your shoulder to the wall behind you. Begin breathing out through your mouth as you return to the front. Pause, then repeat to the right.

5. Continue turning your head from side to side 12–18 times.

WAGGING TAIL TO CALM HEART FIRE

Benefits: I have altered this exercise somewhat to accommodate a seated position. The exercise remains beneficial, however, because the movement still allows the internal organs to massage each other. In addition, the muscles around the spine are exercised, the nervous system is stimulated, and the overall effect is an improved sense of balance. This exercise is similar to *Big Bear Turns from Side to Side* but it is less energetic and requires a return to an upright position when the torso swings back to the center.

1. Because you will be leaning forward and moving your torso from side to side, you may need to shift forward away from the back of your chair. However, your general posture should remain the same—feet shoulder-width apart, head and neck stretched comfortably upward, shoulders pressed downward.

2. Hold your hands high on your thighs. Take a deep breath in through your nose, expanding your diaphragm. As you bend forward over your thighs, begin blowing the breath out through your mouth. Continue blowing outward as you swing your torso to the left, bending your head and looking toward the left side of the room at the same time.

3. Swing back to the center, still leaning over your thighs, and continue on to the right. When you reach the furthest swing to the right, begin lifting back up to the center.

4. Straighten your back and rest for a moment. Repeat the swing, beginning to the right this time. Swing your torso to the left and then return to the upright center position.

5. Continue swinging your torso from side to side with returns to the center for a total of 18 times. Remember to return to the upright center position between each set of pendulum movements and breathe deeply before beginning the swings on the opposite side.

CRANE'S BEAK

Benefits: This is a slow, meditative exercise. Ask your patients to imagine themselves as cranes standing perfectly still on one leg on the bank of a stream, waiting for a fish to swim by. The stillness that the bird exhibits is what they should try to achieve as they move their arms smoothly and gracefully. At the same time, they will benefit by tightening their underarms and strengthening their shoulder muscles. After the previous exercise involving energetic swinging of the torso, this exercise will bring the *qi* back to its resting position in the lower *dan tian*.

1. Check your position on the chair, take a deep breath in through your nose, expanding your diaphragm, and lift both arms to the level of your shoulders.

2. Breathe out and hold your arms stationary. At the point where you are about to breathe in again, begin lifting your arms another five or six inches (13–15cm). Try to coordinate your breathing with your arm movements.

3. As you move your arms upward, bend your wrists and form a bird's beak with your fingers by touching the thumb and other fingers of each hand together (Figure 2.11). Remind your patients that they will still be breathing in through the nose as the arms ascend and form the bird's beak.

4. Lower your arms slowly and gracefully to shoulder level as you blow stale air out through your mouth.

5. Continue lifting and lowering your arms in time with your breathing for at least nine repetitions.

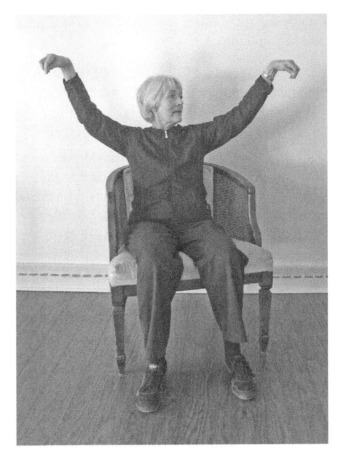

Figure 2.11 Crane's Beak

CRANE FLAPS WINGS

Benefits: Once again, your patients will be moving the *qi* down to the lower *dan tian* and back up through the center of the body to the upper *dan tian.* This exercise should be relaxing, almost hypnotic, in the smoothness of the arm motions. Suggest that your patients concentrate primarily on the movement of their breathing in synchronization with the "flapping wing" motions.

1. Breathe in deeply while you raise your arms to shoulder height. Hold for a moment and then lower your arms, breathing out at the same time.

2. Continue moving your arms to shoulder level and back down as you breathe in and out. Remember to move your arms up and down slowly and smoothly in time with your breathing. Do not form the "bird's

beak" with your fingers. Allow your hands to move naturally with the movement of your arms.

3. Repeat the motion at least nine times and then rest for a moment with your hands on your thighs before beginning the next exercise.

COW LOOKS AT THE MOON BEHIND

Benefits: This exercise is particularly beneficial for the central nervous system, as well as the circulation of blood and energy to the head. It is also said to be good for the kidneys and for strengthening the activity of the eyes, neck, and shoulder muscles. If any of your patients have high blood pressure or hardening of the arteries, recommend frequent use of this exercise.

1. As you breathe in, lift your arms to chest level with the palms facing you.

2. As you breathe out, turn to the left, pushing your hands with the palms facing away from you as far out to the side as possible. Hold this position for a moment.

3. Return to your original position as you breathe in, bringing your arms back in front of your chest, palms facing you.

4. Turn to your right again as you breathe in. Press your arms out to the side, palms facing outward until your arms are stretched as far as possible, without locking your elbows. Hold for a moment and then return to your beginning position.

5. Repeat, alternating sides for a total of 18 times.

LEANING TO THE SIDE TO COOL EXCESS HEAT

Benefits: This exercise relaxes the entire body while reducing tension in the sympathetic nervous system. Use this exercise for your patients when they are particularly stressed.

1. Check your posture again to make sure the small of your back is still against the back of the chair and that your feet remain shoulder-width apart.

2. As you breathe in, raise your right hand over your head, palm facing downward. Lean to the left as far as possible while breathing out (Figure 2.12).

3. Return to an upright position as you breathe in again. Bring your left arm over your head, palm downward, and breathe in.

4. Lean to the right while breathing out. Return to an upright position as you breathe in once again.

5. Continue alternating sides for a total of 18 times.

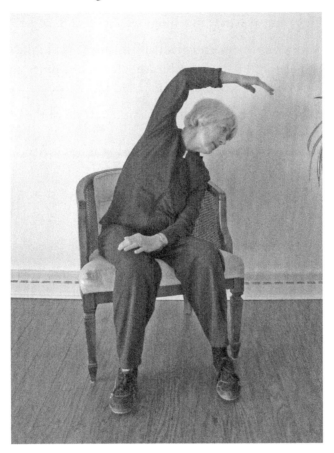

Figure 2.12 Leaning to the Side to Cool Excess Heat

CENTERING QI

Benefits: If the *qi* has become trapped in an area of the body as the result of putting too much emphasis on one exercise or the other, or one side of the body or the other, this exercise will restore the *qi* to its proper balance. Remind your patients that breathing for this exercise is pre-birth or reverse breathing. They should tighten their diaphragms and relax just the lower abdomen when they blow out the stale air from their lungs.

1. Hold your hands palm up just above your lap, fingertips touching (see Figure 2.2, page 27). Breathe in deeply through your nose while contracting your diaphragm. It is only in this one exercise that the diaphragm is *not* expanded during inhalations.

2. As you tighten your diaphragm and abdomen, raise your arms out to the side and up over your head to its center. Your palms are now facing the ceiling, fingers barely touching (see Figure 2.3, page 28).

3. Allow your arms to descend gradually in an arc out to the side. As you do so, exhale until there is no breath left in your lungs and relax just the muscles of your lower abdomen.

4. Return your arms to the original position in front of the lowest part of your abdomen, palms upward.

Level three Qigong exercises

Once again, the opening exercises are designed to warm up the entire body before beginning the Qigong exercises. These basic breathing exercises set the stage for the proper breathing techniques, engaging the *qi* so that it can be released from the lower *dan tian,* and warming up muscles and joints for the movements that follow.

Qigong warm-up exercises

GATHERING QI

Benefits: This warm-up exercise brings the *qi* that may be trapped in other areas of the body into the lower *dan tian.* It is from this area that your patients will pull up energy to the middle *dan tian* and, eventually, into the upper *dan tian,* the repository for mental and spiritual energy.

1. Sit comfortably with your back against the back of your chair, hips tucked slightly under. Make sure your legs are shoulder-width apart. Lift your head as though it is being pulled gently upward by a string attached to the ceiling.

2. Place your right hand over your lower *dan tian*. To be certain that your hand is in the right place, rest your right thumb on your navel. Your hand will then naturally rest on the lower *dan tian*. Place your left hand over your right.

3. Breathe in deeply through your nose and exhale through your mouth. Continue to breathe deeply but naturally for at least one full minute.

STIMULATING QI

Benefits: As your patients swing their arms back and forth, the *qi* from the lower *dan tian* will surge upwards and out to their fingertips. The forward swing lifts the energy to the middle *dan tian* and then out along the arms. This exercise is both soothing and energizing.

1. Check your posture to be sure your feet are still shoulder-width apart and your hips are tucked under so that the small of your back is resting against the back of your chair.

2. Make certain that your arms are on the outside of the arms of your chair at a sufficient distance so you don't bang against the sides as you swing your arms.

3. Begin by swinging your arms backward. Allow both arms to swing forward naturally. Don't try to time your breathing with this exercise. Continue to breathe in through your nose and expel the toxins out through your mouth in your normal breathing rhythm.

4. Begin with at least 36 swings. You may increase the number of swings as you progress.

SPREADING QI

Benefits: This exercise will seem familiar to your patients because it is something we all unconsciously and automatically do when we're cold. By gently slapping their thighs and arms, your patients will increase the circulation in their limbs and distribute the *qi* throughout their bodies.

1. Begin by crossing your arms. Slap your arms gently from the elbows up to the shoulders and back down to the elbows again. Do not try to time your breathing to the slaps.

2. Sit forward on your chair so that you won't hit your arms while you do this exercise. Swing your arms out to the sides and then slap them against your thighs. Continue to breathe naturally—not in time with

your arm movements. You may increase the pressure of your slaps but never to the point of soreness or bruising.

3. Start with 36 slaps on your arms and 36 on your legs. You may build up to a larger number but, as above, never to the point of soreness or bruising.

LIFTING YOUR QI

Benefits: By lifting each leg, your patients will push the *qi* upward into their trunks. As the feet return to the floor, the acupressure points on the soles of the feet are stimulated. See the diagram of foot acupressure points in Appendix B.

1. Sit with your back against the back of your chair again. Tuck your hips underneath you so that the small of your back is supported against the back of your chair. Feet and legs should be shoulder-width apart.

2. Keep your foot parallel to the floor as you lift it to the height of your abdomen or chest (see Figure 2.1, page 26). Change feet and repeat.

3. Continue lifting your legs alternately for at least nine sets with each leg, if possible.

4. Again, you may increase the number of lifts as long as your thigh muscles don't become overly tense. Remember, like Taiji, Qigong should be performed in a relaxed way. Don't allow yourself to become tense as you go through the exercises.

CENTERING QI

Benefits: If the *qi* has become trapped in an area of the body as the result of putting too much emphasis on one exercise or the other, or one side of the body or the other, this exercise will restore the *qi* to its proper balance. Remind your patients that the breathing for this exercise is reverse or pre-birth breathing. When they breathe in, they should tighten their diaphragms and then relax just the lower abdomen when they blow out the stale air from their lungs.

1. Hold your hands palm up just above your lap, fingertips touching (see Figure 2.2, page 27). Breathe in deeply through your nose while contracting your diaphragm. It is only in this one exercise that the diaphragm is *not* expanded during inhalations.

2. As you tighten your diaphragm and abdomen, raise your arms out to the side and up over your head to its center. Your palms are now facing the ceiling, fingers barely touching (see Figure 2.3, page 28).

3. Allow your arms to descend gradually in an arc out to the side. As you do so, exhale until there is no breath left in your lungs and relax just the muscles of your lower abdomen.

4. Return your arms to the original position in front of the lowest part of your abdomen, palms upward.

Qigong exercises

SILK REELING

Benefits: Ask your patients to imagine that their hands are connected to their *qi* by invisible strings so that the *qi* follows the motions of their arms upward to eye level. (Remember, if you encourage each patient to concentrate on the purpose of all these movements, their sessions will be greatly enhanced.) This exercise will strengthen the shoulder and arm muscles and spread energy throughout the upper body and limbs.

1. After checking the position of your feet and that the small of your back is against the back of your chair, press down on your shoulders and lift your head so that it is sitting high and light on your neck.

2. Lift your hands from your lap, leading with your wrists, and bring them upward until your hands are level with your eyes. Breathe in as you lift your arms, letting your hands dangle downward (Figure 2.13).

3. As you breathe out, lower your arms, allowing your hands to return to just above your lap, leading with the heels of your hands.

4. Continue lifting and lowering your hands at least nine times.

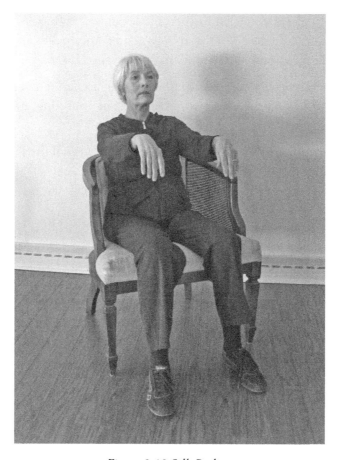

Figure 2.13 Silk Reeling

BEAR TURNS

Benefits: The purpose of this exercise is to stabilize the body, returning the *qi* to the lower *dan tian*. Use this exercise to help your patients strengthen and tighten their upper arms and shoulders. They will notice after a period of time that the backs of their upper arms will have a more sculpted appearance.

1. Inhale deeply and lift both arms, elbows bent, hands level with your ears, palms facing the ceiling (Figure 2.14).

2. Exhale and turn to the left from the waist, keeping your arms in the position described above. Turn as far to your left as you comfortably can.

3. Inhale and return to the center, keeping your arms steady and level.

4. As you exhale, turn to the right as far as possible. Pause for a moment and then, inhaling again, return to the center.

5. Alternating sides, repeat the turning for a total of 18 times if possible. If you experience pain or excessive strain, reduce the number until you build up your strength. Make sure that you do an equal number of turns to each side.

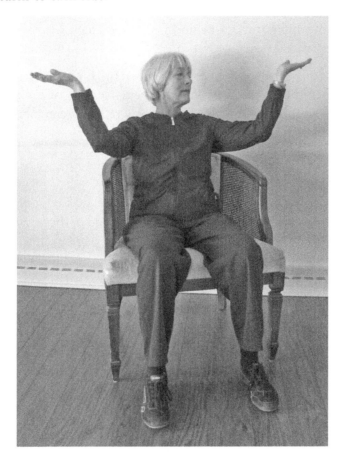

Figure 2.14 Bear Turns (Arm Position)

BEAR PUSHES TO THE BACK

Benefits: Again, this exercise develops the muscles in the shoulders and upper arms. Biceps and triceps both benefit from this exercise without any need for weights or pulleys. Hands should be in the same position as they were in the above exercise (Figure 2.14).

1. Check your posture, then take a deep breath, allowing your diaphragm to expand.

2. Turn to the left from your waist as you exhale and extend your left arm behind you as far back as possible.

3. Inhale as you turn back to the center and then turn to your right, exhaling as you twist from your waist.

4. Press your right arm out behind you, pause, then return to the front, inhaling as you turn.

5. Keep turning from side to side for a total of 18 times if you can. As in the other "Bear" exercises, if you experience pain or excessive strain, reduce the number to a comfortable level but remember to do an equal number of turns to each side.

BEAR PUSHES DOWN

Benefits: As with all the "Bear" exercises, *qi* is sent to the upper body and along the shoulders and down the arms to the hands. These are wonderful tightening and strengthening movements for your patients' muscles in their upper arms and shoulders. In addition, the twisting motions will slenderize their waists while tightening the abdominal muscles.

1. Begin facing forward, chest lifted high, shoulders pressed downward, and legs shoulder-width apart. Remember the small of your back should be resting against the back of your chair.

2. Inhale deeply through your nose and lift your arms with the elbows bent so that your hands are level with your ears. Palms should be facing the ceiling and fingers pointed to the back.

3. Exhale as you turn your upper body to the left, push downward with your left hand, but keep your right hand in the beginning position.

4. Turn back to the center, inhaling as you do so.

5. Twist to the right, exhaling as you turn. When you have turned as far as possible, press your right hand downward alongside your right hip. Pause for a moment and then turn back to the front, inhaling and raising your right hand with the palm upward, level with your right ear.

6. Continue turning from side to side for 18 repetitions. Reduce the number if you experience discomfort or strain, but remember to do an equal number of turns to each side.

BEAR OFFERING

Benefits: Your patients will trim their waists and tighten their abdomens with each twist. Their arms and shoulders will be greatly strengthened and energized.

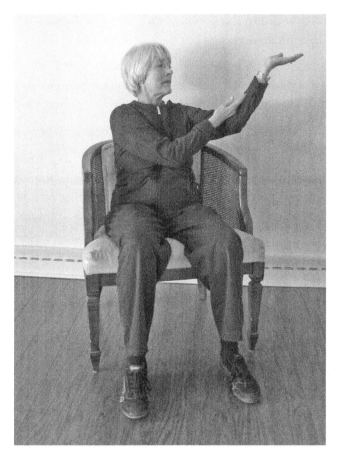

Figure 2.15 Bear Offering

1. Check your posture and then lift both arms so that your hands are just below your breastbone, palms facing up. Take a deep breath.

2. Twist to your left as you begin exhaling. Extend your left arm until it is almost straight and lift it to shoulder height.

3. Stretch your right arm until your right hand, palm upward, is resting on your left forearm (Figure 2.15). Turn back to the center, breathing in as you do so, and return your hands to their original position.

4. Reverse and repeat for a total of 18 times if possible.

BEAR PUSHES SIDE TO SIDE

Benefits: Work on arm and shoulder muscles continues in this exercise. Twisting the waist is beneficial for both the waistline and the abdominal muscles.

1. Begin as you did in the previous exercise, arms below the breastbone, palms up. Inhale deeply.

2. Turn to your left and push both hands out the side as though you were pushing against a wall. Pull your arms back toward your chest and begin inhaling as you return to the center.

3. Take a deep breath, then, as you exhale, begin turning to the right, pushing both arms out to the side as you do so.

4. Continue turning side to side and pushing out to each side for a total of 18 times if you can. If not, reduce the number of repetitions, but make sure you are doing an equal number on each side.

FIRST CROW OF THE ROOSTER

Benefits: Lifting the arms overhead so that the hands are above the *One Hundred Meeting Point* while lifting each leg draws energy from the lower part of the body. In the process, you and your patients are guiding the *qi* up through the middle of the body, connecting the various energies that come together at this acupressure point on the crown of the head.

1. Sit with your feet shoulder-width apart, hands resting on your thighs. Lift your rib cage so that your posture is erect. Press down on your shoulders and hold your head lightly as though it is suspended on a string attached to the ceiling. Tuck your hips under slightly. This will cause the small of your back to rest against the back of your chair, allowing the *qi* to flow freely through the meridians located toward the back of your body.

2. Raise both arms to the side, level with your shoulders, and, at the same time, inhale through your nose, expanding your diaphragm. As you exhale, raise your arms over your head, palms facing, and lift your right leg with the knee bent (Figure 2.16). Hold the position for a moment.

3. Return your arms to shoulder height, timing the movements with the exhalations, and return your foot to the floor.

4. Take a deep breath, expanding your diaphragm and belly. At the same time, bend your elbows, keeping your arms at shoulder height, then press firmly against an imaginary ball between your hands.

5. Exhale, tightening your abdominal muscles and pushing your hands downward as though you are pressing your imaginary ball into a pool of water.

6. Return your hands to your thighs and rest while you complete a cycle of inhale/exhale before beginning the exercise again.

7. Repeat the arm and breathing pattern but change legs for each repetition. In order to guarantee an equal number of leg lifts, repeat the exercise anywhere from six to 18 times.

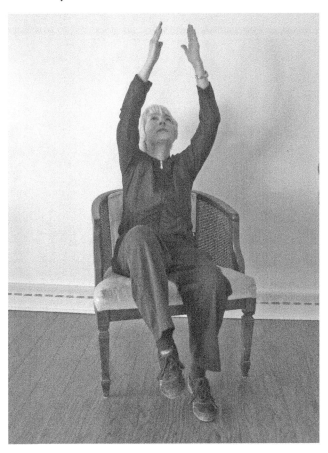

Figure 2.16 First Crow of the Rooster

HOLDING THE SUN

Benefits: This exercise will greatly tighten and strengthen arms and shoulders. Bringing the hands in front of the chest (see Step 3 below) gathers the *qi* into the middle *dan tian*. When your patients' arms are lifted overhead, their energy returns again to that area of confluence of energies at the *One Hundred Meeting Point*. At the end of the exercise, instruct your patients to push the gathered energy back down into the lower *dan tian*.

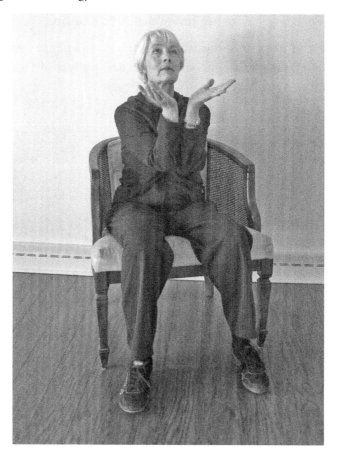

Figure 2.17 Holding the Sun

1. Check your posture again to be sure your back is flat against the back of the chair and that your feet are shoulder-width apart.

2. Raise both arms to shoulder height and inhale, allowing your diaphragm to expand.

3. Exhale and tighten your diaphragm and abdominal muscles as you bring your hands in front of your chest as if pressing against an

imaginary ball (Figure 2.17). Your arm muscles should be taut as though you were trying to squeeze a hard ball between your palms.

4. Take a deep breath, expand your diaphragm, and bring your hands closer together, then turn your hands palms up, pushing the same imaginary ball toward the ceiling.

5. Bend your arms and bring your hands down alongside your ears with the palms facing behind you. When they reach the front of your chest, push your imaginary ball downward as you breathe in deeply.

6. When your hands are just above your lap, release your breath and let your arms dangle alongside your body. Breathe out and relax.

7. Lift your arms to shoulder height again as you breathe in through your nose. Continue this exercise for at least nine repetitions.

INHALING RIVER AND MOUNTAIN

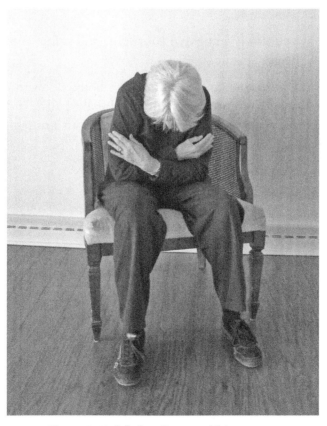

Figure 2.18 Inhaling River and Mountain 1

Benefits: This is the only Qigong exercise in which your patients will be breathing with both the abdomen and the entire chest. These movements will increase the amount of oxygen to muscles, organs, and joints. In addition, the muscles of the entire upper body are strengthened. The action of bending over the legs and then returning to an upright position flexes the back muscles and realigns the spine.

1. Check your posture again and then take a deep breath, expanding your diaphragm.

2. Exhale as you lift your hands slightly above your head, palms facing.

3. Up to this point you have been breathing while tightening and expanding your diaphragm and, to a certain extent, the abdomen. This time when you inhale, expand your entire chest (very gently) as well and move your arms out to the side, palms still facing.

4. Exhale and bend over from the waist and cross your arms, right arm on the inside for women, left arm on the inside for men (Figure 2.18). Pause for a moment.

5. Inhale as you slowly straighten your spine and bring your arms up to shoulder height (Figure 2.19).

6. Move your arms back to the front of your body, elbows rounded. Cup your hands and lower them to your lap. Inhale, pause, and then begin the exercise again by exhaling and raising your arms slightly above your head, palms facing.

7. Repeat all movements at least nine times.

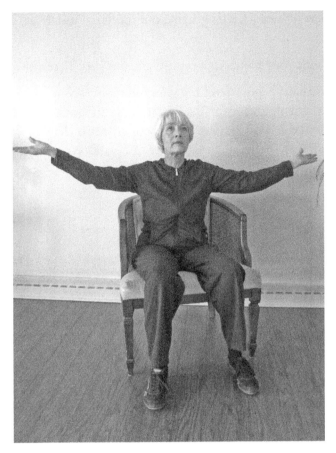

Figure 2.19 Inhaling River and Mountain 2

PUNCHING WITH A STEADY GAZE

Benefits: Use this exercise with your patients to increase their *qi* and for general strengthening. All the muscles of their arms and shoulders will be tightened for a more sculpted look. In addition, it is believed that the act of punching is beneficial for liver functioning and will destroy toxins and allow faster healing after injuries or illness.

1. Begin in the same posture as usual, except this time the small of your back is not against the back of your chair. Your hips should still be tucked slightly underneath you, feet flat on the floor, shoulder-width apart. Make sure that you have enough room between you and the back of your chair so that you can bring your fisted hands to your waist without hitting your elbows against the chair. Now, press your

shoulders down and lengthen your neck as much as comfortably possible.

2. Hold both your hands in a tight fist, palms up. Take a deep breath.

3. As you exhale, begin stretching your right arm forward with a punching motion and tighten your diaphragm and abdomen. Just before your arm reaches its full stretch, twist your hand so that the knuckles are now upward (palm down) (Figure 2.20). Don't lock your arm but keep your elbow bent slightly.

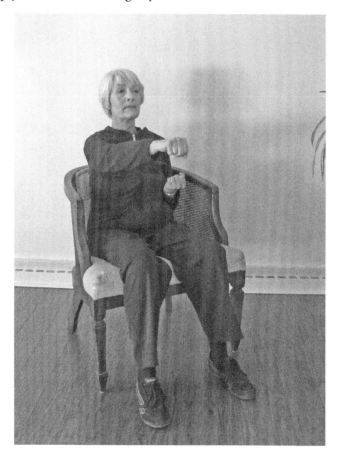

Figure 2.20 Punching with a Steady Gaze

4. As you return your fist to your waist, inhale again, allowing your diaphragm to relax and expand.

5. Punch out slowly but strongly with your left arm, palms up at first, while exhaling and tightening your abdominal muscles. Toward the end of the arm stretch, turn your fist palm down.

6. Return your hand to your waist while inhaling and relaxing your arm muscles. The *yin* or relaxed motion is in the return of the fist to your waist. When you are punching outward, tighten your arm all the way up to the shoulder (*yang*).

7. Continue punching as you gaze steadily forward for as many even-handed repetitions as possible. Your arm muscle should feel tight but not strained. Start with a small number of punches and work up to a larger number of punches as your arms strengthen.

CENTERING QI

Benefits: If the *qi* has become trapped in an area of the body as the result of putting too much emphasis on one exercise or the other, or one side of the body or the other, this exercise will restore the *qi* to its proper balance. Remind your patients that breathing for this exercise is reverse or pre-birth breathing. When they breathe in, they should tighten their diaphragms and then relax just the lower abdomen as they blow out the stale air from their lungs.

1. Hold your hands palm up just above your lap, fingertips touching (see Figure 2.2, page 27). Breathe in deeply through your nose while contracting your diaphragm. It is only in this one exercise that the diaphragm is *not* expanded during inhalations.

2. As you tighten your diaphragm and abdomen, raise your arms out to the side and up over your head to its center. Your palms are now facing the ceiling, fingers barely touching (see Figure 2.3, page 28).

3. Allow your arms to descend gradually in an arc out to the side. As you do so, exhale until there is no breath left in your lungs and relax just the muscles of your lower abdomen.

4. Return your arms to the original position in front of the lowest part of your abdomen, palms upward.

ACUPRESSURE POINTS FOR QIGONG EXERCISES

I have included six basic acupressure points that I believe will enhance your patients' experience with the Qigong exercise sessions. There are, of course, many other very effective acupressure points listed throughout the book. You may use any of the acupressure points listed in the sample lesson or in Chapter 3 on Taiji exercises. These particular points, however, match most perfectly with the internal organs targeted by the Qigong exercises themselves—that is, the spleen, liver, lungs, heart kidneys, and stomach. As usual, I encourage you to experiment to find out what combination of exercises and acupressure points work best for your patients' particular needs.

Spleen Meridian No. 4—Grandfather Grandson

If your patients measure one thumb-width behind the ball in the upper arch of their foot, they will have located this acupressure point. Instruct them to press firmly on this point and hold for 60 seconds.

Benefits: This is a particularly effective point for women to relieve menstrual bloating and abdominal cramps. This point also lessens the symptoms of PMS.

Liver Meridian No. 2—Travel Between

Direct your patients to press their index fingers on the point between the big toe and the second toe on the top of the foot. They should maintain pressure on this area for at least 60 seconds.

Benefits: This is a potent pressure point for the relief of nausea, stomachaches, diarrhea, and headaches.

Kidney Meridian No. 27—Elegant Mansion

This point is located in the depressions directly below the points of the collarbone. Your patients should press firmly on this point and hold for 60 seconds.

Benefits: This is an effective acupressure point for patients who are having breathing difficulties, chest congestion, or coughing from a cold or an allergy. This pressure point also strengthens the immune system and may be used regularly for anxiety and depression.

Lung Meridian No. 10—Fish Border

Ask your patients to turn their hands so that their palms are facing upward. Direct their attention to the center of the pad just below the base of the thumb where they will press firmly with the thumb of their other hand.

Benefits: This is an effective point to relieve coughing and a sore, swollen throat. If your patients' breathing is shallow due to fatigue, stress, or illness, have them press on this point while inhaling deeply and expanding their diaphragms. The diaphragm should contract when the patient breathes out through the mouth. Have your patients use this point several times until their breathing becomes deeper and more relaxed.

Heart Meridian No. 7—Spirit Gate

Direct your patients to run their fingers along the outside of the forearm to the crease at the wrist and then to the little finger side. They should use the thumb from their opposite hand to press on this point for at least 30 seconds.

Benefits: When you notice that a patient is feeling particularly anxious or nervous, or appears to be experiencing periods of forgetfulness, suggest that they use this point for relief.

Pericardium Meridian No. 7—Big Mound

This pressure point is located on the inside of the arm at the middle of the wrist crease. Your patients should press gently but firmly on this point for 30 to 60 seconds.

Benefits: If your patients complain of pain in their wrists or have been diagnosed with tendonitis from repetitious activity, suggest the use of this point. This effective acupressure point can be used often throughout the day.

3
SEATED TAIJIQUAN

Exercises for Health and Fitness

Attain the ultimate emptiness
Hold on to the truest tranquility
The myriad things are all active
I therefore watch their return.

Everything flourishes; each returns to its root
Returning to the root is called tranquility
Tranquility is called returning to one's nature
Returning to one's nature is called constancy
Knowing constancy is called clarity.

Translation of *Tao Te Ching* #16: 1, 2 by Derek Lin
Tao Te Ching: Annotated and Explained (2006)

The beginnings of Taiji

The idea of *tai* first appears in the *Book of Changes* (*Yi Jing*) where the two characters that comprise *tai* refer to the process of change which produces the polar opposites of *yin* and *yang*. The character for *quan* has three possible definitions. It may mean to fight with an empty fist—that is, without weapons—or to collect one's life energies internally, or to balance the *yin* and *yang* energies, or any combination of the three. The usual translation of Taijiquan is "grand ultimate fist," but each of these words also has additional meanings. *Tai* may translate to high, highest, or far in the distance. *Qi* may be used to mean extreme, outermost end or point, a peak, or summit, as well as steam, smoke, breath, life, or energy.

The genesis of the martial art called Taijiquan, however, is not as clear as the meanings of the characters that comprise the words. Conflicting stories abound regarding the origins of this fighting form because of the secrecy surrounding all forms of Chinese martial arts. Most historians, however, credit a man called Zhang Sanfeng with creating the original 13 postures that make up the basic moves used in all Taiji forms.

If Zhang Sanfeng was not the originator of Taiji, he was certainly its most famous teacher and practitioner. His fame was so widespread that an Emperor of the Ming Dynasty (1386–1644) erected a monument to Zhang Sanfeng that still stands today on Wudang Mountain, located in the northwestern area of Hubei Province.

Some historians claim that Zhang lived in the 13th or the 15th century; others that he could not have lived any earlier than the 18th century. In that case, the question arises about the dating of the monument to—at the latest—the 17th century. To whom was this monument dedicated, then, if not to Zhang Sanfeng?

According to Jou, Tsung Hwa (2001) in his book, *The Dao of Taijiquan*, Zhang was born on April 9, 1247 in the Jiangxi Province in southeast China at the Daoist historical site of the Dragon-Tiger Mountain. Zhang was considered to be a "wise man" not just because of his teachings and his healing ability, but also because of his physical appearance. Jou describes Zhang as having an arched back like a tortoise, the tall, slender figure of a crane, and large, round eyes. The Chinese believed that large, round eyes are a sign of intelligence and an assurance of longevity.

As a young man, Zhang passed a test given by the Emperor of the Yuan Dynasty that qualified him for a high government position. According to historical accounts, Zhang accepted the position in spite of the fact that he is said to have had no interest in wealth or power. Perhaps Zhang accepted this post to please his parents for, upon their death, he returned to his home only long enough to give away to relatives all of his possessions and those of his parents. Then, in the company of two young men, he set out in search of a wise man who could teach him the secret of immortality.

For 30 years, Zhang wandered throughout the country, finally settling in the Baozhi Mountains in midwestern China. This mountain range is notable for its three peaks. "San feng" means three peaks in Chinese and thus Zhang came to be known as Zhang Sanfeng or Zhang of the Three Peaks. While living at Baozhi, Zhang met a Daoist by the name of Huolong. Although he studied under Huolong for several years, Zhang was unable to achieve the level of spiritual development he was seeking. Therefore, four years after arriving on Baozhi, Zhang set out again on his quest.

After a period of wandering again through his native land, Zhang settled on Wudang Mountain. Mount Wudang is so magnificent and so beautiful that it has been called the Famous Mountain under Heaven. According to most accounts, it was here that Zhang developed the martial art system known as Taijiquan.

Historians relate a number of stories about the way in which Zhang Sanfeng developed Taiji. Some claim that Zhang dreamt the system and then practiced and taught what he had learned in his dream. Others think that Zhang's experience of witnessing a deadly battle between a crane and a snake was what inspired him to create Taiji. According to this story, Zhang believed the snake was victorious because of its relaxed, circular, and evasive movements and lightning-fast counter strikes. He set about to devise a system for himself and his students that would imitate the movements of the snake as much as possible.

Other writers of Chinese history believe that Zhang evolved his system while watching boxing matches between the monks who lived on Wudang Mountain. Zhang noticed that the monks were off balance during their matches and that the smaller monks were unable to overcome the larger, more muscular men. He concluded that emphasis on outer strength rather than internal power was the reason for the difficulties he had witnessed. His observations led him to consider the principles of Daoism, the Taiji diagram of *yin* and *yang*, and the eight trigrams of the Yi Jing in relationship to exercise and fighting styles.

The Taiji diagram

The Chinese believe that before all things came into being, there was a great void that they call "wuji." This void was empty and full at the same time. It was a nothingness that was full of information and potentiality. *Wuji* then gave rise to *Taiji* which is expressed in the female principle, *yin*, and the male principle, *yang*.

The *Taiji* diagram is a circle that contains two fish-shaped areas: one black, one white. The black section of the circle is *yin* and represents the female principle while the white area is *yang* and symbolizes the male principle. Before the birth of *yin* and *yang*, the circle is *wuji*—that is, it is empty. It is the great void that existed prior to creation.

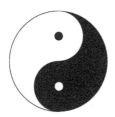

As you look at the *Taiji* diagram shown above, note that the black portion contains a tiny circle of white and the white section holds a tiny circle of black. The significance of each incorporating a portion of the other is that while *yin* and *yang* represent opposite forces, they also each contain a germ of the other. They are understood to be opposed to each other yet unified as a whole. For example, when night (*yin*) reaches its peak, day (*yang*) has, in a sense, already begun. When the sun is at its highest, we can confidently anticipate that night will follow. Some of the activities of these two principles as they seek a balance within the human body are unconscious, driven by the body's own regulating system. Others are the result of our conscious desire to be comfortable. During hot summer months, we seek a spot in the shade and a cool drink, while in the frigid months of winter, a hot drink and a warm fire would be our choices.

Yin is expressed as Mother Earth with her rich soil. It is a womb and a repository for new life or new ideas. It is refreshing and wet like a cool, placid lake, dark and still as the night. The energy or *qi* of *yin* always moves inward and downward and is believed to regulate right-brain activity. *Yang* represents sky and heaven as its energy moves upward and outward. It is the heat of summer, the strength of the summer sun, and a blustery wind. *Yang* is active and acquisitive, denoting the analytical and rational characteristic of left-brain activity. These two elemental forces of nature taken together, then, are in a constant process of evolution.

Keep these two elements in mind as you work your way through the following exercises. It is important to distinguish the *yin* from the *yang* activities. As a rule of thumb, *yin* occurs at that point during which you and your patients are breathing in and your arms or legs are close to your bodies. In many cases, it is when you are almost completely still that you are expressing *yin*. Therefore, when you are moving your arms or legs away from your body and are breathing out, you are expressing *yang*. Don't concern yourself too much with explaining these distinctions at the beginning. When your patients have learned the movements of each exercise sufficiently to go through them smoothly, then turn your attention and theirs to the distinction between the two types of activities. Make sure that the *yin* periods are very relaxed and that your patients know to tense their muscles only during *yang* movements.

Now, check your patients' postures and positions on their chairs and encourage them to take deep, cleansing breaths, then begin the exercises on the following pages. Remember, you can read the instructions directly off the page if you wish, at least until you are comfortable enough with the exercises to explain them without referring to the descriptions.

Exercises for emotional exhaustion

The marvelous inventions that surround us are both a blessing and a curse. They inspire us to greater efficiency and productivity. Because we can multi-task, we feel we must. Bosses and even family members expect it, and we expect it of ourselves.

Some of the people you may be working with fall into the category of people called the "sandwich" generation: middle-aged and employed full-time. These people are still young enough to have dependent children at home, yet old enough to have parents in deteriorating health.

Many college students today are also parents. In an effort to get through school as quickly as possible, they juggle a full load of classes, a part-time job, children, and spouses.

I firmly believe that regular practice of either Taiji or Qigong—or both together—is the best method for combating the stress and fatigue that all of us experience in our lives. My college students find that exams, a heavy load of classes, and their many other responsibilities become tolerable once they learn how to use both these forms of exercise to relieve stress.

Ideally, Taiji should be practiced in the early morning and around sunset in the evening. However, with a hectic schedule that may not always be possible. Unless your patients are truly dedicated, they are unlikely to stick to this type of regimen. Remember, neither you nor they need to adjust your lives completely to benefit from these exercises.

Because Taiji is truly a holistic approach to exercise, the surroundings, music, clothing, and time of day are important to a certain extent. Taiji is customarily performed outdoors in a park. However, whatever you can manage in your work place or your patients' homes will be fine as long as the area is pleasant and reasonably quiet. Pick the most favorable room in the facility where you are working, preferably one with a good-sized window that looks out on a pleasant scene.

To further enhance the mood of the surroundings, you may want to use music to accompany the exercises. If you have a piece of music that you like, use it. But choose carefully. Anything that is too fast, has lyrics, or is too heavy on the rhythm will distract you and your patients from concentrating on the movements and breathing, and may lead you to speed up exercises that are meant to be performed slowly and thoughtfully.

An addition to the room you might consider is a tabletop fountain or waterfall. These are available in many department stores, art galleries, through catalogues, or on the internet. The sound of water is soothing and will aid in the calming of your patients' spirits that we are seeking through the practice of Taiji and Qigong.

Remember to encourage your patients always to wear loose, comfortable clothing, nothing that binds or will constrict them in their movements. Since these exercises are of the seated variety, the question of footwear is of little importance as long as your patients aren't wearing shoes that pinch their feet.

Posture and alignment of the body are so important in properly performing exercises of any kind that I have included a reminder at the beginning of each section here as I did for the Qigong exercises in the previous section.

Double-check the proper posture by imagining for a moment—or try it out before you describe the position to your patients—that you are lying on your back. If your legs are stretched out, there will be a curvature in your back at about the midpoint. If you bend your knees, you are unable to slip your hand between the floor and your back because when you bent your knees, your spine became perfectly flat. This is the posture that you want your patients to have while they are exercising. For our purposes, this means that you will have to draw their attention to tucking under their hips so that their backs will be fully supported by the backs of their chairs. It is best to use chairs that have a solid back that is high enough to support your patients' entire back while they are exercising.

Before you introduce the following exercises, ask your patients to close their eyes for a moment, take several deep breaths, and sink gently into the contours of the chair.

Option one

Exercises	Acupressure points
White Crane	Kidney Meridian No. 27—Elegant Mansion
Push Up Sky/Press Down on Earth	Pericardium Meridian No. 3—Crooked Marsh
The Turtle	Pericardium Meridian No. 6—Inner Gate
Holding Up Sky	Heart Meridian No. 7—Spirit Gate
Centering Qi	Conception Vessel No. 17—Sea of Tranquility
	Governing Vessel No. 20—One Hundred Meeting Point
	Governing Vessel No. 19—Posterior Summit
	Governing Vessel No. 21—Anterior Summit

All breathing in this section of exercises, with the exception of *Centering Qi*, is post-birth breathing—that is, the diaphragm is expanded when breathing in and contracted when breathing out.

WHITE CRANE

Benefits: This exercise releases the energy (*qi*) stored in the middle *dan tian*, alleviating emotional exhaustion.

Posture: Remind your patients to sit with their backs against the back of the chair. Legs should be shoulder-width apart, feet flat on the floor. Make sure their hips are tucked under slightly and shoulders curved inward without hunching. Their heads should be held lightly on their necks as though they were suspended by a string from the ceiling.

Point of origin: Energy (*qi*) is released from the middle *dan tian*.

Visualization for your patients: Imagine that you are squeezing and massaging your internal organs, particularly in the area around the heart.

1. Raise your right hand to the level of your right ear so that your palm is facing forward. Your left hand should be alongside your left thigh, palm pressing down toward the floor.

2. Take a deep breath in through your nose.

3. Turn from your waist as you begin to release your breath through your mouth. At the end of the twist, you should be facing the wall to your left.

4. Bring your right hand down as you lift your left hand (palm forward) to the level of your left ear. Breathe in through your nose as you return to face forward.

5. Continue the rotation to the right and breathe out through your mouth as you do so. As on the other side, the turn is complete when you are facing the wall to your right and your right palm is pressing toward the floor.

6. Reverse and continue repeating from side to side for 18 twists.

PUSH UP SKY/PRESS DOWN ON EARTH

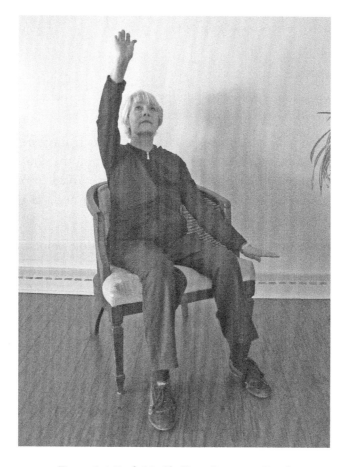

Figure 3.1 Push Up Sky/Press Down on Earth

Benefits: Your patients' energy will be released from the middle *dan tian* so that it is flowing throughout their chest and up and down their arms.

Posture: Remind your patients to sit in the same position as in the previous exercise.

Point of origin: The origin of the energy released by this exercise is, once again, the middle *dan tian.*

Visualization for your patients: Imagine that you are creating a space between the sky and the earth and, by touching both, you are connecting with the energies of each.

1. Raise your right hand and turn your palm toward the ceiling. At the same time, lower your left arm so that your palm is facing the floor

(Figure 3.1). Tighten the muscles of both arms when they are fully extended.

2. As you stretch your arms upward and downward, breathe in deeply through your nose, allowing your diaphragm to expand as fully as possible.

3. Bring both arms level with your diaphragm and blow out your breath slowly through your mouth as you tighten your diaphragm.

4. Breathe in through your nose again as you extend your left arm upwards and your right arm toward the floor.

5. Continue to reverse your arms and repeat the exercise for a total of 18 times.

The Turtle

Benefits: This exercise stretches the neck and shoulder muscles and strengthens the muscles of the abdomen and the diaphragm while releasing emotional stress.

Posture: Your patients should be sitting in the same position as in the previous exercises.

Point of origin: As the muscles of the arms and shoulders are stretched, energy is released from the middle *dan tian*.

Visualization for your patients: Imagine that you are a turtle, poking your head and legs out of your shell and then pulling them back inside again.

1. As you breathe in deeply through your nose, press both arms downward alongside your thighs with your palms facing the floor.

2. Stretch your neck by lifting your head, looking upward toward the ceiling, and pressing down on your shoulders (see Figure 2.6, page 43).

3. Bring your arms, hands fisted, to your chest (at about diaphragm level) and blow out your breath sharply as you bend slightly at the waist.

4. Repeat for a total of nine times.

HOLDING UP SKY

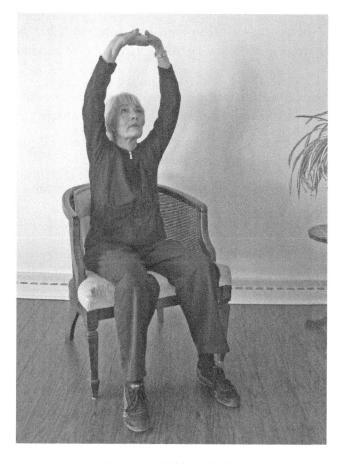

Figure 3.2 Holding Up Sky

Benefits: This exercise circulates the energy through the upper part of the chest while stretching the arm and shoulder muscles.

Posture: Your patients should be sitting in the same position as in the previous exercises.

Point of origin: Once again, the movement of the arms and the pattern of breaths stimulates the energy stored in the middle *dan tian*.

Visualization for your patients: Your hands are touching the heavens and your feet are planted firmly on the earth. You are a conduit of their energies, exchanging and receiving *qi*.

1. Lace your fingers and lift your arms over your head with your palms facing the ceiling (Figure 3.2). As you do so, take a deep breath in through your nose.

2. Swing your arms back down to waist level and blow out your breath through your mouth.

3. Continue to swing your arms up and down while inhaling and exhaling deeply for a total of nine times.

4. On the ninth count upwards, stop and then lean to your right while blowing out your breath. Center your arms again and straighten your back.

5. Take a deep breath in through your nose, then lean to your left and exhale.

6. Continue alternating sides for a total of nine leans. On the last lean, which will be to the right, swing your arms downward in a large arc and swing back upwards to the left, ending with your arms over your head.

7. Take a deep breath again and alternate leans, beginning on the left side.

8. After the nine alternating leans, swing your arms in a large arc and return to an upright position.

9. Repeat the nine arm swings overhead and down to your waist. Remember to keep your hands laced together and your palms toward the ceiling when your arms are above your head.

CENTERING QI

Benefits: This exercise will center the energy and rebalance the body.

Posture: Have your patients sit in the same position as in the previous exercise.

Point of origin: As your patients are engaging in continuous deep diaphragmatic breathing, they are pulling up the energy or *qi* from the lower *dan tian* through the middle *dan tian* and, finally, all the way to the upper *dan tian* that contains their *shen* or mental energy.

Visualization for your patients: Imagine that you are collecting the *qi* and bits of energy from all over your body, returning them to a "neutral" position at the lower *dan tian* so that none will be lost or trapped elsewhere in the body.

In this exercise, the pre-birth breathing method is used—that is, as you breathe in through your nose, contract your diaphragm, and as you breathe out, expand just your lower abdomen.

1. Hold your hands palm up just above your lap, fingertips touching (see Figure 2.2, page 27). Breathe in deeply through your nose while contracting your diaphragm. It is only in this one exercise that the diaphragm is *not* expanded during inhalations.

2. As you tighten your diaphragm and abdomen, raise your arms out to the side and up over your head to its center. Your palms are now facing the ceiling, fingers barely touching (see Figure 2.3, page 28).

3. Allow your arms to descend gradually in an arc out to the side. As you do so, exhale until there is no breath left in your lungs and relax the muscles of your diaphragm and abdomen.

4. Return your arms to the original position in front of the lowest part of your abdomen, palms upward.

Acupressure points to relieve emotional exhaustion

Kidney Meridian No. 27—Elegant Mansion

There are two *Elegant Mansion* acupressure points, one on each side of the breastbone. To help your patients locate these points, ask them to run their fingers along the collarbone until they reach the beginning of their breastbone. Directly below the collarbone on each side there is a hollow area. Instruct your patients to press on both of these indentations with their middle fingers and hold for at least 30 seconds.

Benefits: This potent pressure point relieves breathing difficulties and coughing due to anxiety, stress, or fatigue.

Pericardium Meridian No. 3—Crooked Marsh

Ask your patients to bend one arm and, with their other hand, locate the end of the elbow crease on the inside of the arm. Press and hold for at least 30 seconds on each arm while breathing deeply. Ask them to close their eyes to avoid distractions and concentrate on the in and out movement of their diaphragms and breath.

Benefits: If your patients use this acupressure point, they will experience relief from a nervous stomach and chest discomfort caused by anxiety and fatigue.

Pericardium Meridian No. 6—Inner Gate

Help your patients find this point by measuring two and a half finger-widths from the wrist crease on the inside of their arms. Direct your patients to press on this point firmly but gently for a full minute.

Benefits: When accompanied by deep diaphragmatic breathing, this point will alleviate your patients' nausea, palpitations, and general feelings of anxiety.

Heart Meridian No. 7—Spirit Gate

This pressure point is located on the inside of the arm along the wrist crease directly below the little finger. Ask your patients to press and hold on one side for 30 seconds, then alternate sides. As always, it is helpful if they close their eyes and concentrate on each breath (in through the nose and out through the mouth).

Benefits: You might suggest that your patients use this beneficial pressure point right before bedtime if their minds are racing and they have difficulty falling asleep. *Spirit Gate* is also helpful for general anxiety and cold sweats due to nervousness.

Conception Vessel Meridian No. 17—Sea of Tranquility

Help your patients locate this point by measuring three thumb-widths up from the base of the breastbone along its center. Instruct them to press firmly on this point for a full minute. Repeat as often as necessary.

Benefits: If your patient is prone to panic attacks, suggest the use of this point at the onset of the attack. This pressure point is also useful to relieve hiccups, nervousness, and general anxiety. Sitting in a comfortable chair, breathing deeply, and concentrating on each breath will help them to feel calm.

Governing Vessel Meridian No. 20—One Hundred Meeting Point

Governing Vessel Meridian No. 19—Posterior Summit

Governing Vessel Meridian No. 21—Anterior Summit

All three of these points are on the top of the head and are the most effective antidepressant acupressure points on the body. To help your patients locate the *One Hundred Meeting Point,* ask them to run their fingers to the top of their heads from behind each ear until they find a sizeable indentation. There is another hollow approximately one inch (2.5cm) to the front of the *One Hundred Meeting Point* and another about the same distance to the back of the *One Hundred Meeting Point.* The front point is the *Anterior Summit* and the furthest to the back of the head is the *Posterior Summit.* Have them press firmly with their fingers for a full minute on one or all of these points. They can use these acupressure points as often as necessary.

Benefits: If your patients are having memory problems, suffer from depression, stress-induced headaches, or vertigo, you will want to encourage them to utilize these three points frequently and consistently. Remind your patients to combine the use of these points with deep diaphragmatic breathing.

Option two

Exercises	Acupressure points
An	Kidney Meridian No. 27—Elegant Mansion
Hands Waving in Clouds	Pericardium Meridian No. 3—Crooked Marsh
Fair Lady Works Shuttles	Pericardium Meridian No. 6—Inner Gate
Wrist to Wrist	Heart Meridian No. 7—Spirit Gate
Centering Qi	Conception Vessel No. 17—Sea of Tranquility
	Governing Vessel No. 20—One Hundred Meeting Point
	Governing Vessel No. 19—Posterior Summit
	Governing Vessel No. 21—Anterior Summit

All breathing in this section of exercises, with the exception of *Centering Qi*, is post-birth breathing—that is, the diaphragm is expanded when breathing in and contracted when breathing out.

AN

Benefits: While drawing energy from the middle *dan tian,* your patients are exercising their arm and shoulder muscles and massaging their internal organs.

Posture: Make sure your patients are sitting with their backs against the back of the chair. Legs should be shoulder-width apart, feet flat on the floor. Remind them to tuck their hips under slightly and curve their shoulders inward without hunching. The head should be held lightly on the neck as though it were suspended by a string from the ceiling.

Point of origin: As your patients breathe deeply in each of the exercises, ask them to concentrate on the point in the middle of their bodies slightly below the diaphragm where the middle *dan tian* called *qi* is located. Remember that *qi* is the name of that particular *dan tian* but *qi* (energy) is also stored there. The three *dan tians* are also "cultivation" points for energy, as well as repositories. Remind them to set this disc in motion (with their minds) so that the energy will be released throughout the trunk, arms, and shoulders.

Visualization for your patients: Think of your hands pressing against the molecules of air as you exchange energy with your immediate surroundings. Begin with your elbows bent, hands at shoulder level, palms facing forward.

1. Take a deep breath in through your nose, allowing your diaphragm to expand. At the same time, turn the upper part of your body to the left so that you are facing the wall on that side (Figure 3.3).

2. Blow your breath out slowly through your mouth as you extend both arms until your elbows are almost straight.

3. As you bring your arms back to their original position and turn at your waist to face front, begin inhaling slowly.

4. When you reach the center, facing forward, begin exhaling slowly.

5. Turn from your waist until you are facing the wall to your right and, once again, extend your arms until your elbows are almost straight. At this point your exhalation should be complete.

6. Inhale deeply once more, bringing your arms back to their original position. Continue twisting from left to center, to right, and back to center for a total of 18 repetitions.

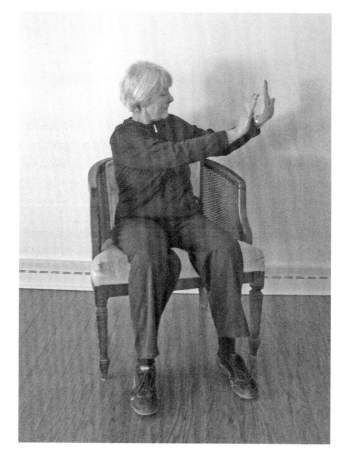

Figure 3.3 An

HANDS WAVING IN CLOUDS

Benefits: The slow, gentle movements of the upper body and arms have a calming effect on the emotions.

Posture: Patients should remain sitting in the same position as in the previous exercise.

Point of origin: The twisting motion of the body from side to side will stimulate the release of energy from the middle *dan tian*.

Visualization for your patients: Imagine that you are brushing wisps of clouds away from in front of your face and abdomen.

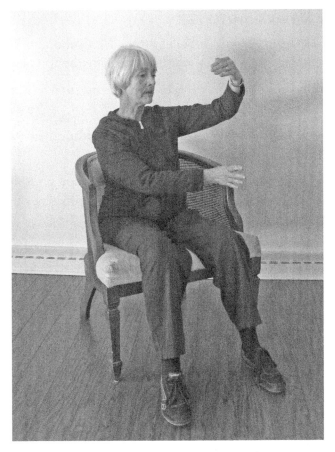

Figure 3.4 Hands Waving in Clouds

1. Bring your left hand level with your eyes, palm facing toward you.

2. Your right hand should be level with your lower abdomen, palm facing the wall to your left so that your wrist is bent slightly back (Figure 3.4). Take a deep breath in through your nose.

3. Twist to your left as far as possible and exhale. Reverse your hands so that your right hand is now level with your eyes and your left is in front of your abdomen.

4. Begin breathing in through your nose as you return to the center position. Don't stop. Continue twisting to your right as you exhale through your mouth.

5. Continue turning at the waist from left to center, to right, and back to center, reversing your hands each time until you have completed 18 twisting motions.

Fair Lady Works Shuttles

Benefits: Once again, energy is being released into the upper part of the body while reducing the waistline and strengthening the arms and shoulders.

Posture: Remind your patients to sit in the same position as in the previous exercises.

Point of origin: As your patients once again twist from their waists, energy is discharged from the middle *dan tian*.

Visualization for your patients: Imagine that you are pressing one hand against a resisting wall of air while your other hand protects your face from the impact of a rush of electromagnetic energy.

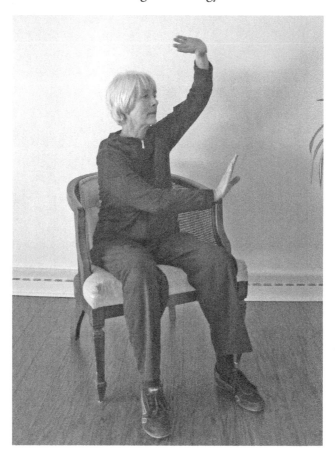

Figure 3.5 Fair Lady Works Shuttle

1. As you turn to your left, raise your left hand in front of your eyes, palm facing outward as though warding off a blow.

2. Thrust your right arm straight in front of you, extending your arm until your elbow is almost completely straight (Figure 3.5).

3. Breathe in as you begin turning to your left and expel your breath when your right arm is fully extended.

4. Inhale again as you return to the center.

5. Breathe out as you turn to the right. Reverse your arms so that your right hand is in front of your eyes and your left pushes forward.

6. Continue changing the position of your hands as you turn from left to right for a total of 18 movements.

WRIST TO WRIST

Benefits: This exercise will strengthen the arms and shoulders, particularly tightening the muscles at the back of the arms. Remind your patients to concentrate on the motions; they will find themselves relaxing if they think only of the push and pull of their arms and the in and out movement of each breath.

Posture: Ask your patients to remain sitting in the same position as in the previous exercises.

Point of origin: This exercise is again an exchange of energy with the air around you and your patients. The middle *dan tian* is stimulated by the movement of the arms and hands.

Visualization for your patients: Imagine that your hands are moving against a wall of air that is pushing back against you. While your movements are relaxed at the beginning, you should tighten your muscles as your arms reach their full extension, without locking the elbow joint.

1. Begin with your left hand held horizontally, palm facing you.

2. Bring your right hand (palm facing away from you, fingers pointed toward the ceiling) to about an inch (2.5cm) behind your left hand so that your wrists are level.

3. Take a deep breath. Then, as you exhale, press both hands forward until your elbows are almost completely straight.

4. Your arm muscles should be loose and relaxed as you begin to extend your arms. As you get closer to the full extension of your arms, however,

tighten your muscles as though you were pushing hard against a solid object.

5. Breathe in as you return your arms to their original position. Hold your breath for a moment and then reverse your hands so that your right hand is in front (held horizontally, palm facing you) and your left hand is behind (held perpendicularly), with the wrists nearly touching, and press forward again as you exhale.

6. Repeat the back and forward motions for a total of 18 times.

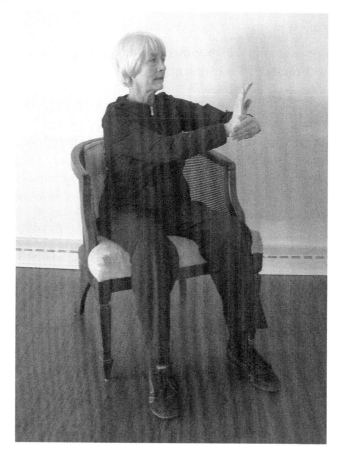

Figure 3.6 Wrist to Wrist

CENTERING QI

Benefits: Centers the energy and rebalances the body.

Posture: Your patients should remain seated as they were for the previous exercise.

Point of origin: Remind your patients to continue with their deep diaphragmatic breathing. The actions in this exercise are pulling the energy or *qi* from the lower *dan tian* through the middle *dan tian,* and, finally, all the way to the upper *dan tian* that contains their *shen* or mental energy.

Visualization for your patients: Imagine that you are collecting the *qi* and bits of energy from all over your body, returning them to a "neutral" position at the lower *dan tian* so that none will be lost or trapped elsewhere in the body.

In this exercise, the pre-birth breathing method is used—that is, as you breathe in through your nose, contract your diaphragm, and as you breathe out, expand just your lower abdomen.

1. Hold your hands palm up just above your lap, fingertips touching (see Figure 2.2, page 27). Breathe in deeply through your nose while contracting your diaphragm. It is only in this one exercise that the diaphragm is *not* expanded during inhalations.

2. As you tighten your diaphragm and abdomen, raise your arms out to the side and up over your head to its center. Your palms are now facing the ceiling, fingers barely touching (see Figure 2.3, page 28).

3. Allow your arms to descend gradually in an arc out to the side. As you do so, exhale until there is no breath left in your lungs and relax just the muscles of your lower abdomen.

4. Return your arms to the original position in front of the lowest part of your abdomen, palms upward.

Acupressure points to relieve emotional exhaustion
Kidney Meridian No. 27—Elegant Mansion

There are two *Elegant Mansion* acupressure points, one on each side of the breastbone. To help your patients locate these points, have them run their fingers along the collarbone until they reach the beginning of the breastbone. Directly below the collarbone on each side there is a hollow area. Direct them to press on both of these indentations with their middle fingers or thumbs and hold for at least 30 seconds. They may use these points whenever they are feeling anxious or having difficulty breathing.

Benefits: These potent acupressure points relieves breathing difficulties and coughing due to anxiety.

Pericardium Meridian No. 3—Crooked Marsh

To use this pressure point, direct your patients to bend one arm and, with the other hand, find the end of the elbow crease on the inside of the arm. They should press and hold for at least 30 seconds on each arm while breathing deeply. Suggest that they close their eyes to avoid distractions and concentrate on breathing and on the in and out movements of the diaphragm.

Benefits: Use this acupressure point for your patients who experience nervous stomachs and chest discomfort caused by anxiety.

Pericardium Meridian No. 6—Inner Gate

Direct your patients to measure two and a half finger-widths from the wrist crease on the inside of their arm. They should press on this point firmly but gently for a full minute.

Benefits: When accompanied by deep diaphragmatic breathing, this point will alleviate nausea, palpitations, and general feelings of anxiety.

Heart Meridian No. 7—Spirit Gate

This pressure point is located on the inside of the arm along the wrist crease directly below the little finger. Your patients should press and hold on one side for 30 seconds, then change arms. As always, suggest that they close their eyes and concentrate on each breath they take in through the nose and expel through the mouth.

Benefits: This is a beneficial point to use right before bedtime. If you know that your patients have trouble falling asleep because their minds are racing or because they are overtired, you might want to show them this acupressure point for use before bedtime. *Spirit Gate* is also helpful for general anxiety and cold sweats due to nervousness.

Conception Vessel Meridian No. 17—Sea of Tranquility

Direct your patients to measure three thumb-widths up from the base of their breastbone along its center to find this acupressure point. Have them press firmly for a full minute. They may use this point as often as necessary.

Benefits: If you have patients who are prone to panic attacks, suggest that they use this point at the onset of the attack. This pressure point is also useful to relieve hiccups, nervousness, and general anxiety. They should find a comfortable chair, breathe deeply, and concentrate on each breath until they begin to feel calm.

Governing Vessel Meridian No. 20—One Hundred Meeting Point

Governing Vessel Meridian No. 19—Posterior Summit

Governing Vessel Meridian No. 21—Anterior Summit

All three of these points are on the top of the head and are the most effective antidepressant acupressure points on the body. To help your patients locate *One Hundred Meeting Point*, have them run their fingers to the top of the head from behind each ear until they find a sizeable indentation. There is another hollow approximately one inch (2.5cm) to the front of the *One Hundred Meeting Point* and another about the same distance to the back of the *Meeting Point*. The front point is the *Anterior Summit*. The point to the back of the *One Hundred Meeting Point* is the *Posterior Summit*. Direct your patients to press firmly for at least a full minute on one or all of these points. They may use these points as often as necessary.

Benefits: If you have a patient who is having memory problems or suffers from depression, stress-induced headaches, or vertigo, you might suggest using these three points frequently and consistently. Remind them to combine the use of these points with deep diaphragmatic breathing while sitting in a quiet area of their home.

Exercises for mental stress

Breath is essential for life, yet we breathe without conscious thought. Unless we make an effort to practice deep breathing, we are all breathing in a shallow way. According to Dennis Lewis, the founder of Authentic Breathing Resources, proper respiration (that is, deep diaphragmatic breathing) may be the single most effective tool for combating asthma, poor digestion, weight gain, sleeplessness, high blood pressure, heart disease, stress, fatigue, and a multitude of other ailments brought about by our modern lifestyle. Deep, conscious breathing cleanses the body and boosts the immune system. How we breathe affects our metabolism because it is *oxygen* that activates the metabolic process that breaks down the fats into carbon dioxide and water, which are then expelled as waste. Of the 42 pints (24l) of fluids that circulate throughout the body every day nourishing and oxidizing the cells, six pints (3.5l) pass through the lymphatic system, cleansing the body of excess proteins, waste products, and fats that would otherwise clog the tissues. The fats that remain in the body are utilized either for energy or are stored for future use. Too much stored fat depletes our energy resources and results in weight gain. For you and me, this means that ignoring the way we breathe jeopardizes our health and practically guarantees that, unless our dietary habits are exemplary, we will gain and retain excess weight.

Healthy breathing also has a profound effect on our emotional state (consider the shortness of breath and tightness in the chest in moments of stress or fear). Deep breathing cleanses not only the body and its many organs and systems but also calms the emotions and heightens our spiritual and intuitive state. Memory and mental clarity can also be vastly improved if we can only teach ourselves to breathe in the right way.

Throughout all these exercises, we are going to concentrate not just on breathing but on *how we breathe* and how to communicate proper breathing to your patients. The basis of Taiji is *non-action* and, for that reason, it is helpful to ask your patients to think of themselves purely as a bundle of bones without flesh or muscles. Though it may seem contradictory, while they are taking action and achieving their desired results, they are doing so in a *non-active* way without straining muscles or stressing the body.

The following exercises specifically target mind and memory. They are designed to alleviate the stress and fatigue which result from our own multitasking lives and the many challenges—physical, emotional and mental—that your patients face every day.

Find a quiet spot to lead your patients through the exercise sessions. Encourage them to concentrate on their breathing, the expansions and contractions of the diaphragm, to stretch their arms as much as possible, and to feel free and to *relax*.

In addition, before you start the sessions with your patients, ask them to center body, mind, and spirit perhaps with a few deep and slow breaths in order to perform the following exercises for their maximum benefit and for the utmost production of fatigue-reducing energy. When you think they are sufficiently relaxed and centered, begin the first exercise.

Option one

Exercises	Acupressure points
Balloon Breathing	Gallbladder Meridian No. 20—Gates of Consciousness
Butterfly	Governing Vessel No. 26—Middle of a Person
Flower Bud Opens	Large Intestine Meridian No. 4—Joining the Valley
Backward Arm Swings	Governing Vessel No. 24.5—Third Eye Point
Centering Qi	Bladder Meridian No. 10—Heavenly Pillar

All breathing in this section of exercises, with the exception of *Centering Qi*, is post-birth breathing—that is, the diaphragm is expanded when breathing in and contracted when breathing out.

BALLOON BREATHING

Benefits: Deep breathing heightens our spiritual and intuitive state. Breathing properly greatly enhances memory, problem solving, right judgment, and mental clarity.

Posture: Remind your patients to begin by sitting with their backs against the back of the chair. Legs should be shoulder-width apart, feet flat on the floor. Their hips should be tucked under slightly and their shoulders curved inward without hunching. The idea here is to keep the *qi* from flowing outward and away from the body. Their heads should be held lightly on their necks as if suspended from the ceiling by a string.

Point of origin: The energy you and your patients release in these exercises is stored in the upper *dan tian*. This storage area contains *shen*, one of the *Three Treasures*. If your patients were to draw a line from the *Third Eye Point* to the back of the head and then another line from the top of one ear straight through the head to the top of the other ear, the mental energy of *shen* would be situated on the intersecting point.

Visualization for your patients: Imagine *shen* as a disc. With your mind, begin rotating that disc until it is spinning very fast. You will notice as the disc spins more and more rapidly that sparks of *qi* or energy begin to shoot out in all directions from the upper *dan tian*. These sparks of energy will reach out to all parts of your head, neck, and shoulders.

1. Hold your hands lightly over your abdomen in the general area of your diaphragm. This will help you to monitor the depth of each breath.

2. Breathe in deeply through your nose and hold the full breath for a second.

3. Blow the stale air out through your mouth until there is no breath left and you must breathe in again.

4. Repeat the deep breaths nine times or longer if necessary, until you feel completely relaxed and energized.

BUTTERFLY

Benefits: Opens the chest to expand the lungs fully.

Posture: Check to be sure your patients are sitting as they were in the exercise above.

Point of origin: The upper *dan tian,* the repository for *shen.*

Visualization for your patients: Imagine your lungs as they expand downward toward your diaphragm, and then outward toward your rib cage.

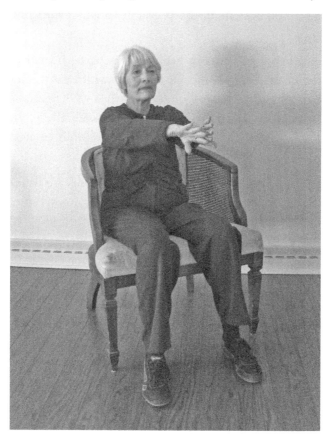

Figure 3.7 Butterfly

1. Begin with your arms bent, hands at waist level, palms up.

2. Move both arms forward at the same time until they are directly in front of your solar plexus.

3. Turn your hands so that they are back to back and continue moving your arms forward until your elbows are straight (Figure 3.7).

4. Press your arms out to the side as though you were propelling yourself through water, and bring them back behind you to their fullest reach.

5. Return your hands to waist level, palms again facing upward.

6. Repeat nine times or until you feel that your lungs have expanded fully and that your chest cavity is open and your fatigue begins to dissipate.

Flower Bud Opens

Benefits: This exercise lifts and opens the rib cage, allowing for a deeper inhalation.

Posture: Remind your patients to begin in their original posture. As they bring their arms above their heads and swing them to the back, make sure they are arching away from the chair.

Point of origin: The point of origin in this exercise is the upper *dan tian*. Help your patients to imagine that their *shen* energy is spinning rapidly now, throwing off sparks of power through the head, upper chest, neck, and shoulders.

Visualization for your patients: Think about your first yawn of the morning. Your chest opens wide as clean, clear air enters your lungs.

1. Begin with your hands in a prayer position (that is, palms pressed together, fingers pointed straight upwards) in front of your solar plexus.

2. Raise your hands above your head, keeping your palms pressed together (see Figure 2.4, page 30).

3. When your elbows are straight, open your arms to the side, sweeping them in an arc to the furthest point possible behind you. As your arms being to circle out to the side, arch your back away from the back of the chair.

4. Return your arms to the prayer position and repeat nine times.

BACKWARD ARM SWINGS

Benefits: This exercise opens the chest cavity, allowing air to flow freely in and out of the lungs. At the same time, your patients are adding strength and tautness to their arm and shoulder muscles while loosening the shoulder joint.

Posture: Remind your patients to maintain their original posture with feet flat on the floor, legs shoulder-width apart, and the small of the back pressed against the back of the chair.

Point of origin: Your patients should continue to concentrate on spinning the disc in the upper middle portion of their heads.

Visualization for your patients: You are exchanging energy with your surroundings. Imagine the molecules of air surrounding you as you push backward, moving your arms through the air's electromagnetic energy.

As in the previous exercises, the breathing method for *Backward Arm Swings* is post-birth breathing. However, do not try to match your breaths with the speed of your arm swings.

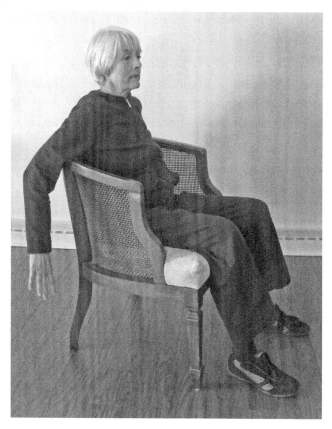

Figure 3.8 Backward Arm Swings

1. Swing your arms backward with a relaxed push as though reaching back to touch a wall behind you (Figure 3.8).

2. Allow your arms to follow through with their natural swing and then push backwards gently again for a total of four sets of nine swings each.

CENTERING QI

Benefits: Centers the energy and rebalances the body.

Posture: Check to be sure your patients are seated as they were in the previous exercise.

Point of origin: As you engage your patients in continuous deep diaphragmatic breathing, let them know that they are pulling up the energy or *qi* from the lower *dan tian* through the middle *dan tian* and, finally, all the way to the upper *dan tian* that contains their *shen* or mental energy.

Visualization for your patients: Imagine that you are collecting the *qi* and bits of energy from all over your body, returning them to a "neutral" position at the lower *dan tian* so that none will be lost or trapped elsewhere in the body.

In this exercise, the pre-birth breathing method is used—that is, as you breathe in through your nose, contract your diaphragm, and as you breathe out, expand just your lower abdomen.

1. Hold your hands palm up just above your lap, fingertips touching (see Figure 2.2, page 27). Breathe in deeply through your nose while contracting your diaphragm. It is only in this one exercise that the diaphragm is *not* expanded during inhalations.

2. As you tighten your diaphragm and abdomen, raise your arms out to the side and up over your head to its center. Your palms are now facing the ceiling, fingers barely touching (see Figure 2.3, page 28).

3. Allow your arms to descend gradually in an arc out to the side. As you do so, exhale until there is no breath left in your lungs and relax just the muscles of your lower abdomen.

4. Return your arms to the original position in front of the lowest part of your abdomen, palms upward.

ACUPRESSURE POINTS TO RELIEVE MENTAL STRESS

Gallbladder Meridian No. 20—Gates of Consciousness

Below the base of the skull, there is a hollow spot between the two large neck muscles on either side of the spine. This is the location of the *Gates of Consciousness* point. Ask your patients to press gently but firmly on this acupressure point for 30 seconds.

Benefits: If you notice that your patients are showing signs of irritability and you suspect this is due to stress and exhaustion, encourage them to use this pressure point often during the day.

Governing Vessel Meridian No. 26—Middle of a Person

The pressure point *Middle of a Person* is located about two-thirds of the way from the upper lip to the base of the nose. Ask your patients to press firmly on this point for two minutes. They may use this point as often during the day as necessary.

Benefits: Although this pressure point is often used to prevent fainting, it is also an effective pressure point for clearing mental processes.

Large Intestine Meridian No. 4—Joining the Valley

Direct your patients to press firmly on the upper part of their hands between the thumb and index finger and directly in front of the bones that join these two digits. This pressure point has many benefits and can be stimulated as often as necessary although it must not be used by pregnant women since it may cause premature contractions.

Benefits: This point is particularly beneficial for the relief of frontal headaches and depression due to stress and fatigue. If you have patients who are having trouble finding the solution to a problem, encourage them to use this point several times during the day to stimulate their creativity.

Governing Vessel Meridian No. 24.5—Third Eye Point

Between the eyebrows there is an indentation at the point where the bridge of the nose meets the center of the forehead. This is the location of the pressure point *Third Eye Point*. Suggest to your patients that they steeple their hands so that both of their index fingers are pressing on the indentation, or they may press just one finger on this spot. Whichever they choose, direct them to press firmly and hold for 30 to 60 seconds.

Benefits: Your patients may find this point helpful for the relief of headaches and eyestrain. This pressure point will aid in relaxing the whole body and easing feelings of nervousness and tension.

Bladder Meridian No. 10—Heavenly Pillar

Direct your patients to run their finger up their necks along the muscle closest to the spine (trapezius muscle). This point is about half an inch (1.25cm) from the base of the skull. They should press on this point for a full minute.

Benefits: Stimulation of this pressure point relieves eyestrain and swelling of the area around the eyes. This point is also useful for alleviating stress, burnout, and mental exhaustion.

Option two

Exercises	Acupressure points
Pull/Push	Gallbladder Meridian No. 20—Gates of Consciousness
Brushing Tree Trunk	Governing Vessel No. 26—Middle of a Person
Plucking Thread	Large Intestine Meridian No. 4—Joining the Valley
Yoga Facelift	Governing Vessel No. 24.5—Third Eye Point
Centering Qi	Bladder Meridian No. 10—Heavenly Pillar

All breathing in this section of exercises, with the exception of *Centering Qi*, is post-birth breathing—that is, the diaphragm is expanded when breathing in and contracted when breathing out.

PULL/PUSH

Benefits: In this exercise, your patients will be pulling the energy (*qi*) from the air around them into their bodies, exchanging waste from their lungs for clear, clean air.

Posture: Make sure that your patients are sitting with the small of their backs against the back of the chair. They should place their feet flat on the floor about shoulder-width apart. Shoulders should be curved slightly inward, but without slouching.

Point of origin: Deep breathing will pull the stored *qi* upward from the lower *dan tian* (three finger-widths below the navel in the center of the body) through the middle *dan tian* (in the center of the body just below the diaphragm) to the upper *dan tian* in the upper center of the head.

Visualization for your patients: As you pull your arms toward your chest, visualize the energy from your immediate surroundings entering your body. As you push your arms forward and breathe out, you are expelling toxic air from the very bottom of your lungs.

1. Begin with your hands resting on your thighs.

2. With palms facing forward, bring your hands toward your abdomen. Move them upward toward your chest while breathing deeply in through your nose. Try to time your breathing and the movement of your hands so that you reach your maximum inhalation at the same time as your hands reach your chest.

3. Push your hands out and forward until your elbows are almost completely straight. Again, match your exhalation to the movement of your hands so that you have expelled all the air by the time your hands reach their furthest extension. Remember not to move away from the back of your chair and to keep the motion relaxed until your arms are almost completely extended.

4. Repeat the arm movements and breaths nine times.

BRUSHING TREE TRUNK

Benefits: This exercise balances the right and left hemispheres of the brain, thereby ridding the mind of distractions, uncertainty, and fatigue.

Posture: Your patients should begin this exercise in the same position as in the previous exercise.

Point of origin: This exercise will stimulate the movement of *qi* from the upper *dan tian,* located in the upper center of the head.

Visualization for your patients: Think about the *qi* as it circulates evenly in and around the right and left hemispheres of the brain, balancing and energizing both creativity and rational thought.

1. Begin by raising your arms until your elbows are straight.

2. Leave your left arm extended while you swing your right arm downward and across your body until your elbow is bent and your arm brushes your thighs. Bend over from the waist so that your chest is directly over the tops of your thighs (see Figure 2.5, page 32).

3. Turn your head so that you are looking up and over your right shoulder.

4. Straighten your upper body as you return your right arm to its upward extension and swing your left arm down and across your body. Look up and over your left shoulder as you bend over your thighs.

5. Repeat nine times on each side for a total of 18 brushes.

PLUCKING THREAD

Benefits: Eye muscles will benefit from following each up and down movement. Additionally, the upper *dan tian* will be stimulated by your patients' concentration on the movements of their hands.

Posture: Your patients should begin in the same position as in the previous exercises.

Point of origin: The origin of the energy flow is from the upper *dan tian.*

Visualization for your patients: Picture yourself pulling threads out of a piece of cloth, one by one. At the same time, you are pulling the energy or *qi* from the lower *dan tian* through the center of your body and up to the level of the upper *dan tian,* the repository for *shen,* your mental energy.

1. Begin with your hands resting on the top of your thighs.

2. Keep your back straight as you lower your right hand between your legs with your fingertips pressed together, then lift your arm (wrist leading) until it is level with your eyes (Figure 3.9).

3. Return your right hand to your right thigh and repeat the same movement as in Step 2 with your left hand.

4. Repeat for a total of 18 up and down movements and remember to follow the movements of your hands with your eyes each time.

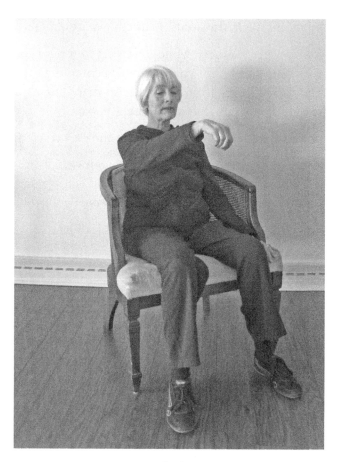

Figure 3.9 Plucking Thread

YOGA FACELIFT

Benefits: This exercise increases circulation to the face and head. The result is a clearer mind, improved skin tone, and the reduction of fine lines and wrinkles.

Posture: Your patients should begin in the same position as in the previous exercises.

Point of origin: The origin of the energy flow is from the upper *dan tian*.

Visualization for your patients: Imagine the increased flow of blood and energy to your brain.

1. Bend over from your hips so that your head is hanging down between your knees. Allow your arms to dangle alongside your thighs.

2. Relax all the muscles of your face. Part your lips slightly. Since your chest is resting on your thighs, you will not be able to breathe deeply from the diaphragm. Instead, breathe lightly through your nose.

3. Remain in this position for one minute if you are able to without becoming lightheaded or dizzy. If the position bothers you, reduce the time to 30 seconds and increase that time gradually as you become more comfortable in this position.

4. As you begin to straighten your back, breathe in and roll yourself upward by straightening your vertebrae from the lowest to the highest, tucking your hips under as you "roll" yourself to the proper sitting position.

CENTERING QI

Benefits: This exercise will center the energy and rebalance the body.

Posture: Your patients' postures should be the same as in the previous exercise.

Point of origin: As your patients engage in continuous deep diaphragmatic breathing, they are pulling up the energy or *qi* from the lower *dan tian* through the middle *dan tian* and, finally, all the way to the upper *dan tian* that contains their *shen* or mental energy.

Visualization for your patients: Imagine that you are collecting the *qi* and bits of energy from all over your body, returning them to a "neutral" position at the lower *dan tian* so that none will be lost or trapped elsewhere in the body.

In this exercise, the pre-birth breathing method is used—that is, as you breathe in through your nose, contract your diaphragm, and as you breathe out, expand just your lower abdomen.

1. Hold your hands palm up just above your lap, fingertips touching (see Figure 2.2, page 27). Breathe in deeply through your nose while contracting your diaphragm. It is only in this one exercise that the diaphragm is *not* expanded during inhalations.

2. As you tighten your diaphragm and abdomen, raise your arms out to the side and up over your head to its center. Your palms are now facing the ceiling, fingers barely touching (see Figure 2.3, page 28).

3. Allow your arms to descend gradually in an arc out to the side. As you do so, exhale until there is no breath left in your lungs and relax just the muscles of your lower abdomen.

4. Return your arms to the original position in front of the lowest part of your abdomen, palms facing upward.

ACUPRESSURE POINTS TO RELIEVE MENTAL STRESS

Gallbladder Meridian No. 20—Gates of Consciousness

Below the base of the skull, there is a hollow spot between the two large neck muscles on either side of the spine. This is the location of the *Gates of Consciousness* point. Instruct your patients to press gently but firmly on this acupressure point for 30 seconds. Then, release the pressure and repeat again for two to three repetitions. Remind them to continue with their deep breathing as they hold their finger on this point.

Benefits: To relieve irritability due to stress and fatigue, encourage your patients to use this pressure point often during the day if you and they feel it is necessary.

Governing Vessel Meridian No. 26—Middle of a Person

The pressure point *Middle of a Person* is located about two-thirds of the way from the upper lip to the base of the nose. Direct your patients to press firmly on this point for two minutes as often during the day as needed if they are experiencing confusion.

Benefits: Although this pressure point is often used to prevent fainting, it is also an effective pressure point for clearing mental processes.

Large Intestine Meridian No. 4—Joining the Valley

This acupressure point is directly in front of the bones that join the thumb and index finger. *Joining the Valley* has many benefits and can be stimulated as often as necessary although it must not be used by pregnant women since it may cause premature contractions.

Benefits: This point is particularly beneficial for the relief of frontal headaches and depression due to stress. If your patients are having trouble finding the solution to a problem, encourage them to use this point several times during the day to stimulate their creativity.

Governing Vessel Meridian No. 24.5—Third Eye Point

Between the eyebrows there is an indentation at the point where the bridge of the nose meets the center of the forehead. This is the location of the pressure point *Third Eye Point*. Suggest to your patients that they steeple their index fingers to press on the indentation, or they may press just one finger on this spot. Whichever they choose, encourage them to press firmly and hold for 30 to 60 seconds.

Benefits: This acupressure point may be used for the relief of headaches and eyestrain. This point will also aid in relaxing the whole body and easing feelings of nervousness, tension, and fatigue.

Bladder Meridian No. 10—Heavenly Pillar

To help your patients find this acupressure point, have them run a finger up their necks along the muscle closest to the spine (trapezius muscle). They should press on the point that is half an inch (1.25cm) from the base of the skull. Time them so they continue pressure on this point for a full minute.

Benefits: Stimulation of this pressure point relieves eyestrain and swelling of the area around the eyes. This point is also useful for alleviating, stress, burnout, and mental exhaustion.

Exercises for physical fatigue

Although the following exercises involve tightening and relaxing the muscles, at no time should there be excessive strain. As in all Taiji movements, relaxation is the key. All the exercises in this book are mainly *mental* exercises—that is, all movement of the energy or *qi* is controlled by the mind. The mind is actively seeking to stimulate the flow of energy in and through the muscles and joints of the body. This is not accomplished by *stressing* muscles or joints but rather by moving this energy through the meridians with the mind.

These meridians include the one that runs up the spine and over the head. The second pathway runs downward from the tip of the tongue back to the perineum. The meridian that circles the waist and the one that runs straight through the center of the body from the perineum to the top of the head are two more pathways that you should draw your patients' attention to during these exercises. The meridians that run up and down the arms and up and down the legs are equally important. Depending upon whether you and your patients are doing upper body exercises or lower body exercises, all of these meridians will be involved in the process.

Five of the junction points are also located in the upper body. There is one junction point directly behind the navel called the *mingmen* and another between the shoulder blades and behind the heart called the *gaohuang*. The third junction point is in the middle of the very top of the head (the *niyuan*), while the fourth is located on the palm (the *laogong*). The fifth junction point is the navel, the *shenque*. These will be points of concentration at different times while you are leading the exercises.

The first set of exercises relaxes and loosens the head, neck, and shoulders. This involves the upper *dan tian* and the last section of the pathway known as the *du mai*, which runs upward along the spine. As they perform the exercises, encourage your patients to concentrate on the beginning of the pathway that returns down the front of the body, called the *ren mai*, and the uppermost part of the channel that rises from the perineum, directly through the center of the body to the top of the head. With the inclusion of shoulder shrugs and drops, ask your patients to visualize both the outer arm meridian at its point of origin and the inner arm meridian at its end. If you have patients who have respiratory problems, whether chronic or temporary, you will want to introduce them to the *gaohuang* junction point located directly behind the heart. A weak heart muscle or palpitations may be due to the absence of sufficient energy flow through this junction.

For the exercise *Bird's Feathered Hand* you should draw your patients' attention to the spatial relationship between their working arm and the air surrounding them. They will increase the strength of their grip through the isometric exercise of closing their hands as though there were a hard ball or some other form of resistance between the fingers and the palm. Bursitis, stiff shoulders or fingers, or pain in the arms or hands may indicate a blockage somewhere along the *yang wei mai* or *yin wei mai*, or possibly at the *laogong* junction.

Wild Horse centers the body when the hands are placed in front of the chest and a deep breath is taken into the lungs. There is an additional benefit in *Wild Horse*. If your patients follow the movement of their hands as they are lifted up and out to the side, they will be exercising their eyes as well as centering their bodies.

The exercise known as *Green Dragon* moves energy from shoulder and ear to the center of the body when the arms are brought in front of the chest. The movement ends with one hand in a knife position and the other brushing the top of the thigh. In this movement, your patients' arms are completely relaxed until they reach the end of the downward motion. At that point, both arms should be stiffened and the breath expelled through the mouth.

Repulse Monkey is a wonderful example of the multiplicity of benefits contained in each of the Taiji exercises. Shoulder muscles are loosened gently by the swing of the working arm. Direct your patients to look over their shoulder as they swing their arm up so the neck muscles are stretched. Following the movement of the arm will exercise their eyes and improve their peripheral vision.

In the *Trunk Rotations* exercise, your patients' attention should again be focused on the placement and activity of the *qi* at the lower *dan tian*. Breathing in and expanding the diaphragm while upright encourages more *qi* activity, resulting in another burst of energy through the system. As an added bonus, hip joints are loosened and abdominal muscles tightened as your patients swing their trunks down and around.

Option two of the exercises in this section primarily works the muscles of the lower body. For *Loosening Knees*, ask your patients to scoot forward slightly on their chairs so they'll have more leverage. The secret here is to relax the muscles and joints of the legs, ankles, and knees until they can approximate a circular motion.

With their back once more against the back of their chairs, ask your patients to begin the *Chair Straddles* by moving one leg at a time out to the side as far as that leg will go, followed by the other leg. Have them hold their legs in place for a second or two and then return them to the front of the chair. Your patients should continue straddling the chair, moving one leg at a time out to the side, each time alternating which leg moves first.

For the exercise *Pushing Up Sky with Foot Rolls*, direct your patients to lift their arms above their heads, palms facing the ceiling while they breathe in. At the same time, they should roll up on the balls of their feet. The latter movement will push the energy through the *yang qiao mai* into the *yongquan* (the junction point on the sole of the foot). As they bring their arms back down alongside their thighs, have them pull their feet back onto the heels. In this movement, they will be returning the energy back up the inside of the leg via the *yin qiao mai* through the *huiyin* and back to the lower *dan tian*.

The purpose of the *Ankle Presses and Circles* exercise is to relax the muscles and tendons in the ankles and feet. Your patients should begin by placing one leg out to the side of the chair, foot balanced on the big toe. As they circle first clockwise and then counterclockwise, remind them to breathe into the movement and imagine that they have "rag doll" ankles—very, very loose. Above all, don't let your patients tense their leg or ankle muscles trying to make a perfect circle with the heel.

For the next exercise, *Bow Stance*, ask your patients to angle themselves on the chair. Have them stretch one leg to the side and back while keeping the foot flat on the floor. To do that, they will have to release the ankle to allow it to bend over the inside of the foot. One way to ensure that the foot remains flat is to *slide* the leg backwards rather than place it behind and to the back. Now have them turn to the other side, bring their legs together, and then repeat the leg slide on the other side. Remind them to alternate legs each time if possible. If they become too tired, have them slide one leg out several times and then switch legs.

Golden Cockerel is a challenge for a sense of balance when practiced standing. Since your patients are seated, however, balance won't be an issue, but there will be a certain amount of pressure on the hip joint and the muscles on the top of the thigh. From the knee down, their working leg should be completely relaxed with their toe pointed downward. Let your patients know that if they use their stomach muscles, they can take some of the pressure off the hip and thigh. This is a good exercise to strengthen their thigh muscles and abdomens as well.

Leg Sweeps Lotus will stretch and relax the leg muscles, while at the same time stimulating the glands in the groin area that are part of the immune system. These glands belong to the lymphatic system that seeks out and destroys harmful bacteria and other foreign agents. Swinging one leg over the other activates the lymph nodes in this area.

Thrust Kicks tighten all the muscles of the leg. As your patients kick each leg forward and blow out their breath, instruct them to tighten their abdominal muscles for added benefit. Remember too, that any movement of their legs stimulates the energy pathways on both the outside and the inside of each leg.

As usual, the exercises always end with *Centering Qi*. It is important to return the energy to its proper location before you and your patients begin another set of exercises or simply as a conclusion to the workout. Once again, you can read the instructions directly off the page if you wish since they are written as though directed toward an individual reading the book.

Option one

Exercises	Acupressure points
Head, Neck, and Shoulders	Conception Vessel No. 12—Center of Power
Bird's Feathered Hand	Bladder Meridian No. 23 and No. 47—Sea of Vitality
Wild Horse	Lung Meridian No. 1—Letting Go
Green Dragon	Stomach Meridian No. 36—Three Mile Point
Repulse Monkey	Bladder Meridian No. 48—Womb and Vitals
Trunk Rotations	Bladder Meridian No. 54—Commanding Middle
Centering Qi	Governing Vessel No. 16—Wind Mansion

All breathing in this section of exercises, with the exception of *Centering Qi*, is post-birth breathing—that is, the diaphragm is expanded when breathing in and contracted when breathing out.

HEAD, NECK, AND SHOULDERS

Benefits: This exercise relaxes the muscles of the neck and realigns the cervical vertebrae.

Posture: Have your patients begin by sitting with their backs against the back of the chair. Their legs should be shoulder-width apart, feet flat on the floor. Remind them to tuck their hips under slightly and curve their shoulders slightly inward without hunching. They should hold their heads lightly on their necks as though their heads were suspended by a string from the ceiling.

Point of origin: Since you and your patients are targeting physical fatigue with these exercises, it is important to bring energy from the lower *dan tian* up and through the middle and upper *dan tians*. The neck is considered to be the link between the body and the mind. By concentrating on the movement of the *qi* as it rises through the center of the body, your patients will be able to ease the tension between mind and action that may be causing stiffness and pain in shoulder and neck muscles.

Visualization for your patients: Imagine that your neck muscles are as supple as an infant's and that your head is a light ball perched on a flexible stalk.

Warning: Be sure to thoroughly check your patients' medical history before you have them do this exercise if you think they may have had surgery on their necks or a serious injury to that area.

1. Breathe in while your head is upright.

2. Lower your head gently to your chest while breathing out.

3. Return your head to center, breathing in again, and lower it gently backwards as you breathe out. Repeat nine times, counting the forward and backward motion as one.

4. Now, let your head drop down toward your right shoulder. Return your head to center and then relax your neck muscles as you lower your head to your left shoulder.

5. You will finish with your head tilted to the right. Circle your head down to your chest and then back to the left. Do not lean your head backwards while circling.

6. Continue circling your head for a total of nine times.

7. Lean your head over your left shoulder, then to your right, and so on for a total of nine times.

8. Again, beginning on the left side, circle your head from left to chest to the right shoulder for a total of nine times.

9. Look over your right shoulder and turn your eyes in the same direction as though you were trying to look at someone standing behind you. Now, glance over your left shoulder. Continue alternating side to side nine times.

10. Look over your left shoulder and tilt your head so that you are looking up into the corner where the wall and ceiling meet. Repeat the same movement to the right and continue alternating for a total of nine times.

11. Raise your shoulders toward your ears. Allow them to drop abruptly. This is a particularly good exercise for stiff shoulders. If, however, you experience pain when dropping your shoulder, lower them gently instead. Repeat the shoulder lifts and drops nine times.

12. Circle your shoulders backward, letting your arms dangle loosely by your sides.

13. Breathe into the shoulder joint to make the rolling motion easier. Repeat the shoulder rolls nine times.

14. Now, circle your shoulders forward. Remember to relax your arms completely.

15. Continue circling for a total of nine times.

BIRD'S FEATHERED HAND

Benefits: This exercise will strengthen the muscles of your patients' forearms and hands, increasing the power of their grip.

Posture: Check to be sure your patients are still sitting correctly.

Point of origin: The energy begins in the torso, moves up to the shoulders, and then down the outside of your patients' arms through their middle fingers to the juncture point, the *laogong*. The *qi* then returns to the shoulder by way of the meridian on the inside of the arm (*yin wei mai*).

Visualization for your patients: Imagine molecules of air passing between your fingers. As you close each hand, picture those molecules as solid matter that you must press flat as you make a tight fist.

1. Fist your hands loosely in front of your shoulders.

2. Extend your right arm out to the side and, as you do so, keep the arm and fingers relaxed (Figure 3.10).

3. Now, open your fingers like a bird's individual feathers spread when in flight.

4. Close your hand in a fist again, as tightly as you can. Hold for a moment and then relax your grip and the muscles of your arm as you return that arm to the original position in front of your shoulder.

5. Repeat with the left hand. Don't forget that your hand and arm muscles should be relaxed at all times until the arm is completely extended. At that point, close your fist as tightly as you can and tense your arm muscles. Relax all the muscles again with your hand in a loose fist as you return your hand to the shoulder.

6. Repeat nine extensions to each side for a total of 18 repetitions.

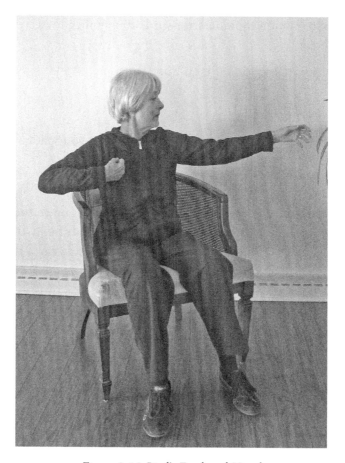

Figure 3.10 Bird's Feathered Hand

WILD HORSE

Benefits: This exercise centers the *qi* and stretches the muscles along the sides of the trunk and the arms.

Posture: Your patients' posture should remain the same as in the previous exercise. If you notice that they are moving away from the back of the chair or slumping as you lead them from exercise to exercise, take time to help them readjust their positions.

Point of origin: Once again, your patients should be concentrating on spinning the disc of the lower *dan tian* to stimulate the flow of physical energy throughout the body.

Visualization for your patients: As you hold the imaginary ball in front of you, picture the energy caught between your hands.

1. Hold your hands, palms facing, with your right hand on top, palm down, and your left hand on the bottom, facing up. Your hands should be as far apart as they would be if you were holding a basketball. Your right hand will be at the level of your solar plexus, and your left hand at the level of your lower abdomen.

2. Now, bring your left hand from below your right hand and raise it to the side and up to eye level. Meanwhile, the right hand moves down and to the side with the palm facing the floor.

3. Return to the center and reverse your hands so that your left is now on top and your right is underneath. Make sure that your hands are as far apart as if you were holding a basketball.

4. Raise your right arm to the side and up to eye level as the left arm presses down and to the side. Return to the center, reversing your hands again.

5. Repeat for a total of 18 times, nine times per side, alternating each time.

Green Dragon

Benefits: This exercise will energize the upper part of the body as it strengthens shoulder and upper arm muscles and trims the waist.

Posture: Ask your patients to remain seated in the same position as in the previous exercises.

Point of origin: Make sure your patients breathe deeply and that they concentrate on releasing the energy once again from the lower *dan tian*.

Visualization for your patients: Picture yourself holding a light bag. Swing it over your shoulder easily and gently. Even though you are not straining, the muscles, particularly at the back of your arms, will become taut and sculpted.

1. Bring both arms over your right shoulder, muscles very relaxed. Your left hand should be level with your shoulder, your right hand in line with your right ear.

2. Lower your hands slowly so that the left crosses your chest, brushing your left thigh, ending palm downward to the side of that thigh (Figure 3.11). Tighten the muscles of your arm as you lower it.

3. The right hand ends in front of the upper chest, held perpendicular to your body so that your palm is facing left. This is the "knife hand" position in Taiji. By the time your hand reaches the front of your chest, the muscles of your right arm should be taut.

4. Reverse your original position so that your right hand is almost cupping your left shoulder and your left hand is level with your left ear.

5. Sweep both arms downward again.

6. Your right hand will finish alongside your right thigh and your left in the knife position in front of your chest.

7. Repeat the swings over your shoulders for a total of 18 times.

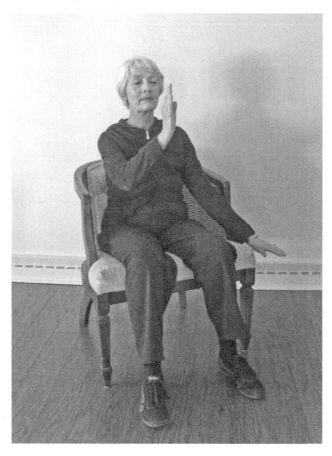

Figure 3.11 Green Dragon

REPULSE MONKEY

Benefits: Repetition of this movement will bring a considerable amount of energy to the hands and will help to rebalance the body.

Posture: Ask your patients to remain seated in the same position as in the previous exercises.

Point of origin: Have your patients concentrate their thoughts on the lower *dan tian* from which we all derive our physical energy.

Visualization for your patients: Imagine the electromagnetic energy passing between your two palms as you move one hand over the other.

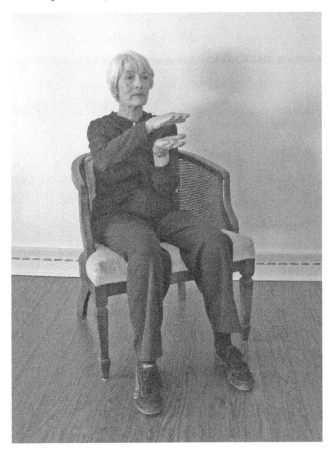

Figure 3.12 Repulse Monkey

1. Hold your left hand at face level with the palm facing upward.

2. Swing your right arm back, following the motion with your eyes by turning your head to look over your shoulder.

3. Now, sweep your arm forward and over your shoulder so that your right hand will pass over your left about one to two inches (2.5–5cm) above it (Figure 3.12).

4. Bring your right hand past your left hand, facing slightly forward, fingers curled a bit.

5. Turn your right hand palm up and swing your left arm behind you as you turn your head to follow the motion.

6. Bring the left hand over the right (palms will be facing) without touching your hands together.

7. Slide the left hand forward, palm slightly raised, fingers curled.

8. Repeat the exercise, alternating hands, for a total of 18 times.

TRUNK ROTATIONS

Benefits: This is an all-purpose exercise. The movements loosen the hip joints, stretch the muscles of the back, and reduce the waistline by tightening the abdomen.

Posture: Make sure your patients remain seated in the same position as in the previous exercises.

Point of origin: All of the movement comes from the lower abdomen and the hips, thereby directly stimulating the lower *dan tian*.

Visualization for your patients: Imagine the destruction of fat particles as they are broken up by the energy flowing through your trunk.

1. Begin again with your hands resting on your thighs.

2. Breathe in deeply, expanding your diaphragm.

3. Circle your trunk to the left, brushing the tops of your thighs with your chest (Figure 3.13). Blow out your breath and tighten your abdomen.

4. Continue circling to the left for a total of nine times, returning to the upright position each time.

5. Take a deep breath again and this time circle counterclockwise or to the right, blowing out your breath as you bend over your thighs.

6. From the center, circle your trunk to the right or counterclockwise, breathing in before you begin. Exhale as you reach the lowest point of the arc. Then, tighten your abdomen as your chest brushes the tops of your thighs.

7. Repeat nine times in each direction for a total of 18 repetitions.

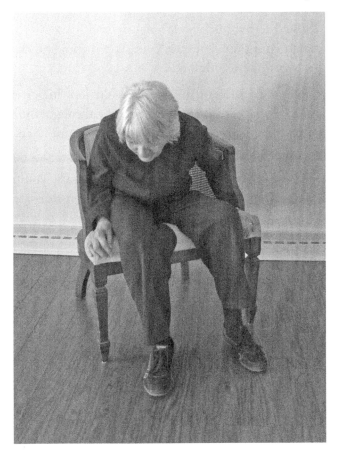

Figure 3.13 Trunk Rotations

CENTERING QI

Benefits: This exercise centers the energy and rebalances the body.

Posture: Ask your patients to remain in the same posture as in the previous exercise.

Point of origin: As you and your patients engage in continuous deep diaphragmatic breathing, you are pulling up the energy or *qi* from the lower *dan tian* through the middle *dan tian* and, finally, all the way to the upper *dan tian* that contains your *shen* or mental energy.

Visualization for your patients: Imagine that you are collecting the *qi* and bits of energy from all over your body, returning them to a "neutral" position at the lower *dan tian* so that none will be lost or trapped elsewhere in the body.

In this exercise, the pre-birth breathing method is used—that is, as you breathe in through your nose, contract your diaphragm, and as you breathe out, expand just your lower abdomen.

1. Hold your hands palm up just above your lap, fingertips touching (see Figure 2.2, page 27). Breathe in deeply through your nose while contracting your diaphragm. It is only in this one exercise that the diaphragm is *not* expanded during inhalations.

2. As you tighten your diaphragm and abdomen, raise your arms out to the side and up over your head to its center. Your palms are now facing the ceiling, fingers barely touching (see Figure 2.3, page 28).

3. Allow your arms to descend gradually in an arc out to the side. As you do so, exhale until there is no breath left in your lungs and relax just the muscles of your lower abdomen.

4. Return your arms to the original position in front of the lowest part of your abdomen, palms upward.

Acupressure points to relieve physical fatigue

Conception Vessel Meridian No. 12—Center of Power

Help your patients locate this point by measuring three finger-widths below the base of the breastbone along the midline of the body. Encourage them always to use gentle pressure on this point and never hold for longer than two minutes. It is best for them to use this point when their stomachs are fairly empty.

Benefits: This is a potent point for the relief of indigestion, nausea, and constipation.

Bladder Meridian No. 23 and No. 47—Sea of Vitality

Help your patients find this point by measuring two (No. 23) and four (No. 47) finger-widths from their spines at the level of their waists. Both of these points will be awkward spots to reach and to press for your patients with just their fingers. Pick out one set of the points first and then ask your patients to fist their hands at these spots and lean back against the back of their chairs. This will ensure greater pressure and therefore quicker relief from pain and discomfort in their lower backs.

Benefits: The *Sea of Vitality* is a pair of useful points for the relief of lower backaches, general fatigue, and postpartum discomfort.

Warning: Do not use this point for a patient who has broken or fractured bones or disintegrating discs. Chronic back problems such as herniated discs *might* benefit from gentle pressure at this point if approved by a physician.

Lung Meridian No. 1—Letting Go

To help your patients find this point, ask them to measure four finger-widths upward from the armpit crease and one finger-width away from the shoulder. Suggest that they press firmly and hold for a full 60 seconds.

Benefits: Use this pressure point for patients who are suffering from chest congestion and tension, coughing, or asthma.

Stomach Meridian No. 36—Three Mile Point

On the outside of the kneecap and four finger-widths below the bottom of the knee there is a good size depression. Check to see if your patients have the right area by asking them to flex and point their feet. They will know they're in the right spot if they feel a muscle flexing as they move their feet. Direct your patients to press firmly on this acupressure point for at least 60 seconds. They may use this point as often as necessary.

Benefits: This is an excellent acupressure point to relieve gas, bloating, stomachaches, and poor digestion.

Bladder Meridian No. 48—Womb and Vitals

Help your patients find this point by directing them to measure one to two finger-widths to the outside of the sacrum—that is, the large bony mass at the base of the spine. Make sure that they are pressing at the midway point between the top of the hipbone and the base of the buttock. Have your patients press firmly on this point for a full minute. To ensure that your patients are able to press firmly enough, have them fist their hands at the *Womb and Vitals* point and lean back against their fists and the back of the chair.

Benefits: Suggest this point to any of your patients who have a lower backache or are suffering from sciatica, pelvic tension, or hip pain.

Bladder Meridian No. 54—Commanding Middle

This point is located at the back of the knee in the middle of the crease. Direct your patients to press firmly with their thumbs behind each knee and hold for a full minute.

Benefits: This is an excellent point to use for your patients who have a sore or stiff back, sciatica, or arthritis of the knees, back, or hips.

Governing Vessel No. 16—Wind Mansion

Your patients can find this acupressure point by running their fingers down from the base of their skulls until they feel the large hollow where the spine meets the head. Have them press gently for a full minute or until they feel some relief.

Benefits: Use this point for your patients who complain of a stiff neck, nasal congestion, or a headache.

Option two

Exercises	Acupressure points
Loosening Knees	Conception Vessel No. 12—Center of Power
Chair Straddles	Bladder Meridian No. 23 and No. 47—Sea of Vitality
Pushing Up Sky with Foot Rolls	Lung Meridian No. 1—Letting Go
Ankle Presses and Circles	Stomach Meridian No. 36—Three Mile Point
Bow Stance	Bladder Meridian No. 48—Womb and Vitals
Golden Cockerel	Bladder Meridian No. 54—Commanding Middle
Leg Sweeps Lotus	Governing Vessel No. 16—Wind Mansion
Thrust Kicks	
Centering Qi	

All breathing in this section of exercises, with the exception of *Centering Qi* and *Golden Cockerel*, is post-birth breathing—that is, the diaphragm is expanded when breathing in and contracted when breathing out.

LOOSENING KNEES

Benefits: This exercise provides an excellent method for lubricating and relaxing knee and ankle joints.

Posture: Direct your patients to sit forward on their chairs with feet and knees together. Have them bend over slightly from the hips and place their hands on their knees, cupping the joints.

Point of origin: Once again, your patients will be stimulating the flow of energy from the lower *dan tian*. This time, however, remind them to direct the flow downward along the meridians of the legs to the knees and ankles.

Visualization for your patients: Imagine that your knees are loose and pliable. The action of circling your knees by pressing with your hands promotes the flow of synovial fluid around the knee cap, refreshing and lubricating the moving surfaces of the joint.

1. Use your hands to rotate your knees to the right or counterclockwise. Try not to move your body any more than is absolutely necessary. Isolate your arms and legs by relaxing your shoulder and hip muscles so that your whole body is not rotating. Repeat the rotations nine times.

2. Reverse the direction so that you are now circling your knees to the left or clockwise. Repeat nine times.

3. Push your knees gently apart while keeping your feet together. Relax your hands and allow your knees to close back together. Repeat for a total of nine times.

CHAIR STRADDLES

Benefits: This exercise stretches and strengthens the inner thigh, replacing flab with muscle.

Posture: Direct your patients to begin by sitting with their backs against the back of the chair. Legs should be shoulder-width apart, feet flat on the floor. Remind them to tuck their hips under slightly and curve their shoulders slightly inward without hunching, and to hold their heads lightly on their necks as though their heads were suspended by a string from the ceiling.

Point of origin: Because you are working the lower part of the body in these exercises, instruct your patients to direct the flow of energy downward from the lower *dan tian* into the hips and thighs.

Visualization for your patients: Imagine that you can see through your skin to the thigh muscles underneath. Feel the muscles lengthen and then contract, breaking up fat particles and tightening the muscles.

1. Breathe in, expanding your diaphragm as you slide your right leg first, then your left leg, out to the side of your chair (Figure 3.14).

2. Blow out your breath as you press both legs back as far as you can. Releasing your breath will relax the muscles, allowing for a wider stretch. Hold the straddle position for ten seconds.

3. Continue alternating the lead leg for a total of 18 stretches, pressing and holding the straddle for ten seconds each time.

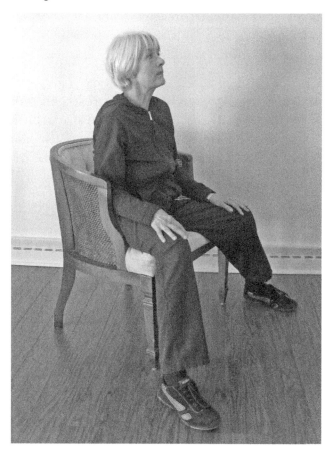

Figure 3.14 Chair Straddles

PUSHING UP SKY WITH FOOT ROLLS

Benefits: This exercise stretches the whole body while strengthening the feet and loosening the ankle joints.

Posture: Instruct your patients to sit in the same position as in the previous exercise.

Point of origin: Once again, the motion of the lower *dan tian* is accelerated to release the stored *qi*. Your patients' minds must direct the flow of that energy downward to the soles of their feet and upward to the top of their heads.

Visualization for your patients: Imagine that you are a conductor of electromagnetic energy, bringing the energy of the earth up through your body to the air around and above your head and downward again to return the energy to the ground beneath your feet.

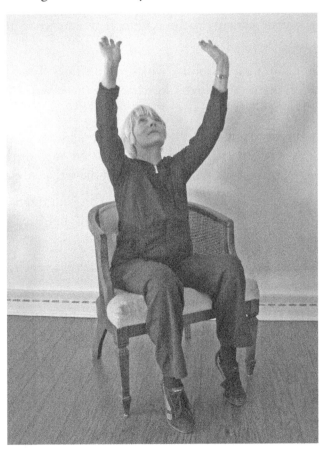

Figure 3.15 Pushing Up Sky with Foot Rolls

1. Roll your feet up onto the balls while pressing your arms toward the ceiling, palms up (Figure 3.15).

2. Take a deep breath as you lift your arms and roll your feet, expanding your diaphragm but keeping your back against the back of the chair.

3. Now, bring your arms down alongside your thighs, palms toward the floor while simultaneously rolling your feet back onto the heels. You should feel a good pull along the calf muscles at the back of your legs.

4. Repeat the entire sequence for a total of nine times.

ANKLE PRESSES AND CIRCLES

Benefits: This exercise will first loosen your patients' ankle joints in a relaxed way. With their feet off the floor, their thigh muscles will be tightened, stretched, and toned. Ankle presses strengthen both feet and ankles.

Posture: Check your patients to be certain they are sitting in the same position as in the previous exercise.

Point of origin: Your patients' minds will direct the flow of energy from the lower *dan tian* through their thighs, knees, down their lower legs, and into their ankles and feet.

Visualization for your patients: Picture the strength and tautness of your thighs, feet, and ankle muscles during the pressing and lifting exercises. Imagine your ankles are soft and rubbery during the relaxed exercises.

1. Begin with your hands resting comfortably on your thighs. Rock your feet back and forth from the heels to the balls and back to the heels without tension. Repeat nine times.

2. Lift your feet off the floor, thighs stretched straight. Flex and point your toes nine times.

3. Now, circle one foot at a time, to the inside. Reverse and circle one foot at a time to the outside. Each foot will complete 18 circles, nine in each direction.

4. Return your feet to the floor. Press up firmly on the ball of your right foot. Hold for a moment and then rock back on your heel and hold again. Change to your left foot and repeat the sequence of ball to heel and back to ball. Do nine sets of foot rolls on each foot for a total of 18 ball-to-heel rolls.

5. Slide your right leg over the side of the chair. While resting on the big toe, circle your heel nine times in one direction and then nine times in the other (Figure 3.16).

6. Change legs and repeat the ankle circles with the left foot and ankle for a total of nine times in each direction.

7. Lift both feet off the floor again, legs out straight, and wag your feet for about ten seconds to loosen the ankle joints.

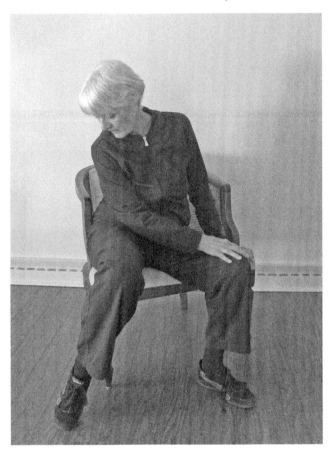

Figure 3.16 Ankle Presses and Circles

Bow Stance

Benefits: The *Bow Stance* is a gentle method for trimming and toning leg muscles.

Posture: Your patients should be sitting in the same position as in the previous exercise.

Point of origin: Encourage your patients to use their minds to direct the flow of energy from the lower *dan tian* down their thighs through their lower legs, ankles, and feet. As they return their legs to the beginning position, the energy will return once again to the lower *dan tian*.

Visualization for your patients: Imagine the fat particles as they break apart and flush away. Feel your thigh muscles as they become stronger and tighter.

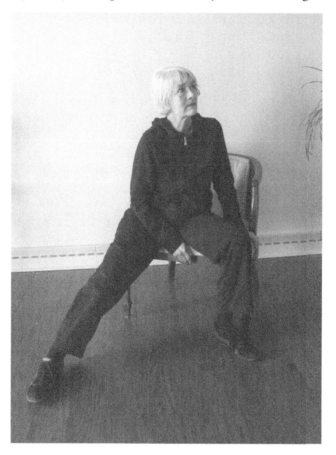

Figure 3.17 Bow Stance

1. Turn to your left so that you are angled on your chair. Keep your legs together.

2. Breathe in deeply and then exhale as you stretch your right leg out to the side of your chair and as far behind you as possible (Figure 3.17). Keep your foot flat on the floor. To make this movement easier at first, start with your foot flat on the floor and then slide it along the floor

until your leg is as straight as you can manage. Hold for at least ten seconds.

3. Reverse directions so that you are angled to the right on your chair. Repeat the same slide along the floor with your left leg until your knee is as straight as possible. Hold for ten seconds.

4. Do nine leg stretches on each side so that you complete 18 total stretches.

GOLDEN COCKEREL

Benefits: Repetition of this movement trims and tones the leg muscles, particularly those of the thigh. Since it is the abdominal muscles that are used in the leg lifts, the abdomen itself is firmed and the belly tightened.

Posture: Your patients should be sitting in the same position as in the previous exercise.

Point of origin: The movement of the legs stimulates the flow of energy from the lower *dan tian.*

Visualization for your patients: Imagine the *qi* flowing along the meridian on the outside of your leg as you lift. The *qi* then returns up the inside of your thigh as you return your foot to the floor.

In this exercise, the pre-birth breathing method is used—that is, as you breathe in through your nose, contract your diaphragm, and as you breathe out, expand just your lower abdomen.

1. Begin with your right leg. Lift your leg with your knee bent to abdomen or chest level. Breathe in, lift your rib cage, and tighten your diaphragm. Concentrate on the action of the muscles of your abdomen and the muscles on the top of your thigh. By tightening these sets of muscles, your thigh is pulled upward toward your torso.

2. Hold your working leg in position for the duration of the inward breath and then lower your leg slowly as you release your breath and relax your diaphragm. Always lower your leg more slowly than you lifted it. This will increase the tension on the thigh muscles, trimming and toning your thighs more quickly.

3. Now, change to your left leg. Repeat the breath in, the lift of your rib cage, and the contraction of your diaphragm as you raise your leg toward your abdomen or chest. Remember to lower your leg more

slowly than you lifted it and in time with the exhalation of your breath and relaxation of your diaphragm.

4. Continue alternating the lifts until you have completed nine lifts with each leg for a total of 18 lifts.

LEG SWEEPS LOTUS

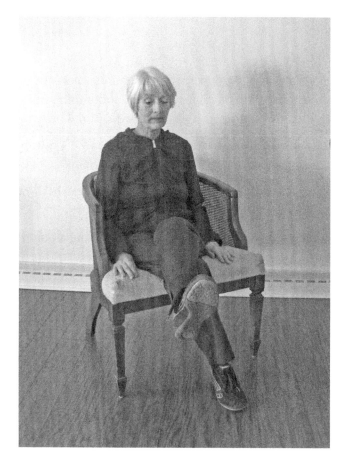

Figure 3.18 Leg Sweeps Lotus

Benefits: This exercise benefits the entire body by stimulating the lymph glands in the groin to produce lymphocytes—that is, the small white blood cells that carry out the activities of the immune system. The movements limber up the hips, reducing daily stress on this weight-bearing joint as well as strengthening the joint to prevent injury.

Posture: Once again, your patients should be sitting in the same position as in the previous exercise.

Point of origin: The lower *dan tian* is again stimulated to release stored energy to the lower abdomen, hips, legs, and feet.

Visualization for your patients: Imagine the *qi* or energy moving through and around the lymph glands, increasing the flow of trillions of blood cells that scrub away toxins from your entire system.

1. Sweep your right leg up and across your left thigh. Return your right leg to the beginning so that it is in line with your right shoulder, flat on the floor.

2. Lift your left leg and swing it up and across your right thigh (Figure 3.18). Return your left leg to its original position.

3. Continue alternating legs until you have completed nine sweeps with each leg for a total of 18 sweeps.

Thrust Kicks

Benefits: This exercise will strengthen the muscles of your patients' thighs and stretch their Achilles tendons and calf muscles.

Posture: Make sure your patients are still seated in the same position as in the previous exercise.

Point of origin: By lifting and stretching their legs, your patients will be bringing the energy in the lower *dan tian* to their lower abdomens and down their legs.

Visualization for your patients: Imagine the tightening action of your thigh muscles as the energy flows downward, invigorating your legs and feet.

1. Lift your right leg with the knee bent. Stretch your leg until your knee is as straight as possible. Point your toe toward the ceiling and hold the extended position for at least ten seconds. Slowly lower your foot to the floor.

2. Lift your left leg with the knee bent and again straighten out your knee as much as possible. Remember to keep your foot flexed so that your toes are pointed toward the ceiling (Figure 3.19).

3. Repeat the exercise alternating legs until you have completed nine leg stretches with each leg. If your muscles cramp when you are holding your leg out straight, allow your thigh to remain on the chair to relieve the pressure on the muscles. After a time you will be able to lift the leg off the chair and hold it out straight.

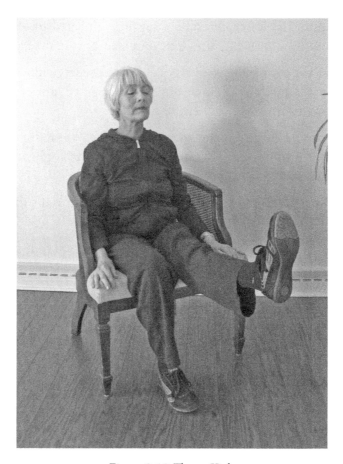

Figure 3.19 Thrust Kicks

CENTERING QI

Benefits: This exercise centers the energy and rebalances the body.

Posture: Ask your patients to remain in the same posture as in the previous exercise.

Point of origin: As you and your patients engage in continuous deep diaphragmatic breathing, you are pulling up the energy or *qi* from the lower *dan tian* through the middle *dan tian* and, finally, all the way to the upper *dan tian* that contains your *shen* or mental energy.

Visualization for your patients: Imagine that you are collecting the *qi* and bits of energy from all over your body, returning them to a "neutral" position at the lower *dan tian* so that none will be lost or trapped elsewhere in the body.

In this exercise, the pre-birth breathing method is used—that is, as you breathe in through your nose, contract your diaphragm, and as you breathe out, expand just your lower abdomen.

1. Hold your hands palm up just above your lap, fingertips touching (see Figure 2.2, page 27). Breathe in deeply through your nose while contracting your diaphragm. It is only in this one exercise that the diaphragm is *not* expanded during inhalations.

2. As you tighten your diaphragm and abdomen, raise your arms out to the side and up over your head to its center. Your palms are now facing the ceiling, fingers barely touching (see Figure 2.3, page 28).

3. Allow your arms to descend gradually in an arc out to the side. As you do so, exhale until there is no breath left in your lungs and relax just the muscles of your lower abdomen.

4. Return your arms to the original position in front of the lowest part of your abdomen, palms upward.

ACUPRESSURE POINTS TO RELIEVE PHYSICAL FATIGUE

Conception Vessel Meridian No. 12—Center of Power

Help your patients find this acupressure point by having them measure three finger-widths below the base of the breastbone along the midline of the body. Remind them always to use gentle pressure on this point and never hold for longer than two minutes. It is best for your patients to use this point when their stomachs are fairly empty.

Benefits: This is a potent point for the relief of indigestion, nausea, and constipation.

Bladder Meridian No. 23 and No. 47—Sea of Vitality

You and your patients can find this point by measuring two (No. 23) and four (No. 47) finger-widths from the spine at the level of the waist. Both of these points are awkward spots for your patients to reach and to press with just their fingers. Choose one set of the points first and then instruct your patients to fist their hands at these spots and lean back against the back of their chairs. This will ensure greater pressure and therefore quicker relief from pain and discomfort in their lower backs. Hold for 30 to 60 seconds for each set of acupressure points.

Benefits: The *Sea of Vitality* is a useful point for the relief of lower backaches, general fatigue, and postpartum discomfort.

Warning: Do not use this point with your patients if they have broken or fractured bones or disintegrating discs. Chronic back problems such as herniated discs *might* benefit from gentle pressure at this point if recommended by a physician.

Lung Meridian No. 1—Letting Go

To help your patients find this point, direct them to measure four finger-widths upward from the armpit crease and one finger-width away from the shoulder. They should press firmly and hold for a full 60 seconds.

Benefits: Recommend this acupressure point for your patients who complain of chest congestion and tension, coughing, or asthma.

Stomach Meridian No. 36—Three Mile Point

Ask your patients to measure four finger-widths below the bottom of their knees where they will find a good size depression. Check to see if your patients have the right area by having them flex and point their feet. They will know they're in the right spot if they feel a muscle flexing as they move the foot. Suggest that they press firmly for at least 60 seconds. They may use this acupressure point as often as necessary.

Benefits: This is an excellent point for relieving gas, bloating, stomachaches, and poor digestion.

Bladder Meridian No. 48—Womb and Vitals

To help your patients find this point, have them measure one to two finger-widths to the outside of the sacrum—that is, the large bony mass at the base of the spine. Make sure that they are pressing at the midway point between the top of the hipbone and the base of the buttock. Direct them to press firmly and hold for a full minute. To ensure that they are able to press firmly enough, have them fist their hands at the *Womb and Vitals* point and lean back against their fists and the back of the chair.

Benefits: Recommend this point if you have a patient suffering from lower backache, sciatica, pelvic tension, or hip pain.

Bladder Meridian No. 54—Commanding Middle

This point is located at the back of the knee in the middle of the crease. Direct your patients to press firmly with their thumbs behind each knee and hold for a full minute.

Benefits: This is an excellent point to use for a patient who has a sore or stiff back, sciatica, or arthritis of the knees, back, or hips.

Governing Vessel Meridian No. 16—Wind Mansion

Help your patients locate this acupressure point by running their fingers down from the base of the skull until they find the large hollow where the spine meets the head. Suggest they press gently on this point for a full minute or until they feel some relief.

Benefits: Recommend this point if you have a patient with a stiff neck, nasal congestion, or a headache.

Exercises for relaxation

One of my favorite poems was written by Deng Ming-Dao in which the author describes a cat sitting in the sun, a turtle sitting on a rock lifting her head upward to the sun, and a frog seated on a lily pad. The question the author asks is "Why aren't people so smart?"

Why do we consider quiet time to be such an unimportant or, worse, "peculiar" practice? Meditative stillness need not be considered a burden or a task to be discharged when we would rather be doing something else. Like dogs and cats and frogs and turtles, we too need a time of stillness, every bit as much as we need the air we breathe and the food we eat.

If we accept the Taoist belief that the universe is a seamless web, a totality of existence where no thing and no one stands alone, then we must be open to receive the lessons nature teaches us. Whether we look to agriculture as the early Taoists did, to our own gardens, or to the animals that inhabit our homes, we see a pattern of life that we would do well to imitate. Why can't we be like the dog lying in the grass, the turtle stretching its neck to receive the warmth of the sun's rays, or the frog resting peacefully on the lily pad?

In this portion of seated Taiji, and following up on the thoughts expressed above, encourage your patients to strive for peace of mind and soul, and a total relaxation of the body. Here, they can recharge their batteries, recenter their energy, and rebalance their whole selves, mind, body, and spirit. For a few moments, at least, you and they will experience what it means to just *be*.

You will recognize some of the exercises in this section because they were included in previous sections. Others will be new to you and to your patients. Options one and two include more exercises than does option three. This arrangement will give you some flexibility for those instances when you have less time to devote to working with your patients. All three sections include self-massage and acupressure points.

The only equipment required in acupressure is your patients' own fingers and hands. Through acupressure and self-massage, they can learn to be proactive with their own health. For many common, everyday aches and pains, they will be able to rely on themselves to relieve the symptoms and rebalance their bodies. They can use acupressure on themselves and you can use it for your patients safely and repetitively. This form of therapy requires no particular training other than experimentation by you and your patients to determine which points will be the most useful for their needs. With a little practice, you and they will become adept at finding the exact spots on the skin and will learn how much pressure is appropriate in each case.

The regular use of these acupressure points has a number of health benefits. Acupressure balances the internal environment of the body while counterbalancing changes in the immediate surroundings. In addition, frequent use of the proper acupressure points will reduce tension and increase circulation.

The points listed below and throughout the other exercise sections have been in use for many centuries to treat ailments and relieve aches and pains by blocking the pain gates, or neurochemicals, of the brain. Pressing on particular points allows the *qi* or energy to flow unimpeded through the meridians and systems of the body. Stimulating blood and lymph flow makes the body more resistant to disease and can aid in weight loss by balancing the digestive system and reducing the stress that sometimes contributes to overeating and weight gain.

Self-massage, though not quite as relaxing as massage therapy performed by someone else, is still an efficient way to reduce tension and stress without the time and expense necessary for a visit to a professional therapist. Massage, much like acupressure, stimulates the flow of blood and lymph to all parts of the body. Massage also fires up the nerve receptors on the skin. Moving the hands over arms, shoulders, face, and legs will cause the blood vessels to dilate, thereby facilitating the flow of blood. Pressing against the skin reaches the muscles underneath, causing those muscles to expand and contract while assisting the circulation of lymph. The gentle stretching action of the muscles during a massage keeps the surrounding tissues elastic, making them more supportive and less inclined to injury during physical activity.

Oxygen capacity can increase after massage by as much as 10 to 15 percent. The body's secretions and excretions are also increased by massage, along with a boost to the metabolic rate. When the metabolic rate increases, the body's cells absorb and utilize the fuel provided by food at a faster rate which, in turn, reduces the absorption and storage of fat. By rubbing along the surface of the skin, nerve endings are stimulated and the flow of nourishing blood is increased to the internal organs.

Regular massage (whether self-massage or that given by a massage therapist) enhances the condition of the skin by stimulating the oil and sweat glands. Increasing the production of sweat clears toxins from the body and the surface of the skin. The additional output of oils from the sebaceous glands lubricates and softens the skin.

Eighty percent of all disease is stress-related. Frustration, insecurity, and fatigue cause the overproduction of the hormones norepinephrine and hydrocortisone by the adrenal gland. Too much norepinephrine and hydrocortisone constrict the blood vessels (vasoconstriction), reducing the flow of blood through the veins and arteries. This constriction makes the heart work harder, breathing is more rapid and shallow, and the digestive processes slow considerably. The result can be migraines, hypertension, depression, or indigestion. Massage, along with the use of appropriate acupressure points, reduces stress, increases circulation, facilitates digestion, and opens the chest cavity and lungs for deeper, more healthful breathing.

Remember: You can read the instructions directly off the page if you wish since they are written as though directed toward individuals using the book themselves.

Option one

Exercises	Acupressure points
Balloon Breathing	Stomach Meridian No. 3—Facial Beauty
Butterfly	Stomach Meridian No. 2—Four Whites
Brushing Tree Trunk	Bladder Meridian No. 10—Heavenly Pillar
Centering Qi	Stomach Meridian No. 6—Jaw Chariot
Self-massage	Triple Warmer Meridian No. 15—Heavenly Rejuvenation
Massage of face and head	Triple Warmer Meridian No. 4—Active Pond
Massage of thymus	Pericardium Meridian No. 7—Big Mound
Massage of shoulders and arms	Pericardium Meridian No. 6—Inner Gate
Meditative relaxation	

All breathing in this section of exercises, with the exception of *Centering Qi*, is post-birth breathing—that is, the diaphragm is expanded when breathing in and contracted when breathing out.

BALLOON BREATHING

Benefits: Deep breathing heightens the spiritual and intuitive state. Your patients' memory, problem solving, right judgment, and mental clarity in general are greatly enhanced once they have learned to breathe properly.

Posture: Make sure that your patients are sitting with their backs are against the back of the chair. Legs should be shoulder-width apart, feet flat on the floor. Remind them to tuck their hips under slightly and curve their shoulders inward without hunching. The idea here is to keep the *qi* from flowing outward and away from the body. They should hold their heads lightly on their necks.

Point of origin: The energy to be released in these exercises is stored in the upper *dan tian*. The energy stored in this area is called *shen* and is one of the *Three Treasures*. If you were to draw a line from the *Third Eye Point* to the back of the head and then another line from the top of one ear straight through your head to the top of the other ear, *shen* would be stored on the intersecting point. Help your patients locate this point so they are aware of what is happening during this exercise.

Visualization for your patients: Imagine *shen* as a disc. With your mind, begin rotating that disc until it is spinning very fast. You will notice as the disc spins more and more rapidly that sparks of *qi* or energy begin to shoot out in all directions from the upper *dan tian.*

1. Hold your hands lightly over your abdomen in the general area of your diaphragm. This will help you to monitor the depth of each breath.

2. Breathe in deeply through your nose and hold the full breath for a second.

3. Blow the stale air out through your mouth until there is no breath left and you must breathe in again.

4. Repeat the deep breaths nine times or longer if necessary, until you feel completely relaxed.

BUTTERFLY

Benefits: Opens the chest to expand the lungs to their fullest extent.

Posture: Check your patients to be sure they are seated properly as in the exercise above.

Point of origin: The upper *dan tian,* the repository of *shen.*

Visualization for your patients: Imagine your lungs as they expand both downward toward your diaphragm and outward toward your rib cage.

1. Begin with your arms bent, hands at waist level, palms up.

2. Move both arms forward at the same time until they are directly in front of your solar plexus.

3. Turn your hands so that they are back to back, and continue moving your arms forward until your elbows are straight (see Figure 3.7, page 104).

4. Press your arms out to the side as though you were propelling yourself through water, and bring them back behind you to their fullest reach.

5. Return your hands to waist level, palms again facing upward.

6. Repeat nine times or until you feel that your lungs have expanded fully and that your chest cavity has been opened as much as possible.

BRUSHING TREE TRUNK

Benefits: Balances the right and left hemispheres of the brain, thereby ridding the mind of distractions and uncertainty.

Posture: Direct your patients to begin in the same position as in the previous exercise.

Point of origin: This exercise will stimulate the movement of *qi* from the upper *dan tian* which is located in the upper center of your patients' heads.

Visualization for your patients: Think about the *qi* as it circulates evenly in and around the right and left hemispheres of the brain, balancing and energizing both creativity and rational thought.

1. Begin by raising your arms until your elbows are straight.

2. Leave your left arm extended while you swing your right arm downward as you bend from the waist, then across your body until your elbow is bent and your arm brushes your thighs (see Figure 2.5, page 32).

3. Turn your head so that you are looking up and over your right shoulder.

4. Return your right arm to its upward extension and swing your left arm down across your body while bending over from the waist. Look up and over your left shoulder.

5. Repeat nine times on each side for a total of 18 brushes.

CENTERING QI

Benefits: Centers the energy and rebalances the body.

Posture: Check your patients' posture to be sure they are sitting as they were in the previous exercise.

Point of origin: As your patients engage in continuous deep diaphragmatic breathing, they are pulling up the energy or *qi* from the lower *dan tian* through the middle *dan tian* and, finally, all the way to the upper *dan tian* that contains their *shen* or mental energy.

Visualization for your patients: Imagine that you are collecting the *qi* and bits of energy from all over your body, returning them to a "neutral" position at the lower *dan tian* so that none will be lost or trapped elsewhere in the body.

In this exercise, the pre-birth breathing method is used—that is, as you breathe in through your nose, contract your diaphragm, and as you breathe out, expand just your lower abdomen.

1. Hold your hands palm up just above your lap, fingertips touching (see Figure 2.2, page 27). Breathe in deeply through your nose while contracting your diaphragm. It is only in this one exercise that the diaphragm is *not* expanded during inhalations.

2. As you tighten your diaphragm and abdomen, raise your arms out to the side and up over your head to its center. Your palms are now facing the ceiling, fingers barely touching (see Figure 2.3, page 28).

3. Allow your arms to descend gradually in an arc out to the side. As you do so, exhale until there is no breath left in your lungs and relax just the muscles of your lower abdomen.

4. Return your arms to the original position in front of the lowest part of your abdomen, palms upward.

Self-massage

Massage of face and head

Benefits: Relaxes all muscles and returns body, mind, and spirit to a state of calm.

Posture: Your patients' positions on their chairs should be the same as in the previous exercises. If you find they have altered their positions, take a moment to help them readjust. Remind them to pay particular attention to their feet, legs, and back.

Point of origin: Ask your patients to concentrate on spreading *qi* from the lower *dan tian* throughout their bodies.

Visualization for your patients: Picture the energy moving through your body, bringing calm to your mind and emotions.

1. Rub your palms briskly together until they are warm. Close your eyes and place your warm palms over them. Hold for about 30 seconds.

2. Then, steeple your hands and press against the *Third Eye Point* (that is, the indentation between your eyebrows above the nose bone). If you are congested due to allergies or a cold, use the middle finger of your left hand to press the *Third Eye Point* and the middle finger of your right hand to press on the top of your head where a baby's soft spot is (the *Posterior Summit Point*). Hold for 30 seconds.

3. Pinch your eyebrows gently between your thumb and index fingers. Beginning at the inside corner, slide your fingers along your brows to the outside corners. Keep your eyes closed while you concentrate on relaxing your eye muscles. Repeat the sliding motion nine times.

4. Massage your temples with your fingertips upward and outward for a total of nine times.

5. Massage from the base of your nose along the cheekbone to the outside edge of your eyes. If your sinuses are congested, you will feel immediate relief as you run your fingertips along the side of your nose. Repeat the motion nine times.

6. Using your fingertips, again massage from the base of your jaw on both sides of your mouth, upward and outward. Don't bear down too hard but exert enough pressure to bring the healing blood to the surface of your skin. Again, massage this area at least nine times.

7. Give your ears a thorough going-over with your fingertips. It is believed that every part of the body is represented at various points on the ears.

8. Using both thumbs, rub along the mastoid process at the back of the ears. Do not do this exercise if you are wearing a hearing aid.

9. Press your middle finger at the base of the skull at the pressure point called the *Wind Mansion*. Hold your finger there for 20 to 30 seconds.

10. Tap with your fingertips (using both hands) from the base of the skull just above the *Wind Mansion* through the center of the head. Keep your hands close together until you reach the hairline. Separate your hands and continue tapping along each side of your head and return to the center again.

11. Using the heel of your hand, press on the frontal bones. Move your hands to the side of your head and press on the temporal bones on each side. Move your hands back and toward the top of your head. Press against the bones covering the parietal lobe. Move your hands

back still further until you feel the ridge at the base of the skull. Press in this area for a few seconds.

12. Now, relax your arms while you circle your tongue, mouth closed, clockwise and then counterclockwise. Circle your tongue nine times in each direction.

13. Press—don't grind—your front teeth together. Work your jaw muscles strongly by pressing the back teeth together on one side. Change to the other side and repeat for nine times on each side.

14. Clasp your hands together behind your head. Push against your hands using your neck muscles. Repeat nine times and then bring your hands down to your thighs and rest.

Massage of thymus

Benefits: Considered the youth gland in ancient China, this area was stimulated to ward off illness and to keep the body vigorous and youthful.

Posture: Your patients' posture should remain the same as it was in the previous exercises.

Point of origin: Though the *qi* or energy is initially brought up from the lower *dan tian,* in this exercise your patients will want to concentrate their efforts on the middle *dan tian* and the upper *dan tian* in order to calm their emotions and quiet their minds.

Visualization for your patients: As you massage the thymus, imagine that you are releasing immune-producing energy throughout your entire body, destroying harmful bacteria and the free radicals that cause aging.

1. Attached to your collarbone and directly above the breastbone is a V-shaped bone. Half a finger-width below the V you will feel a small depression. The thymus gland is directly behind this hollow.

2. Press your index or middle finger firmly on this spot and hold for at least 30 seconds. You may also circle your finger on the indentation clockwise and then counterclockwise for the same amount of time.

Massage of shoulders and arms

Benefits: Much of our daily stress results in pain and tension in the shoulders. When your patients massage their shoulders, the warmth and motion of their hands will relax the muscles and bring fresh blood to the surface of the skin, firming and toning the arms.

Posture: Your patients' posture should remain the same as in the previous exercises.

Point of origin: Direct your patients' attention to the area between the middle and the upper *dan tians*. This is the area they will be stimulating in this exercise to calm their spirits and relax their minds.

Visualization for your patients: Picture a spray of warm, soothing water cascading down your shoulders and arms, washing away the tensions of the day.

1. With your opposite hand, brush your fingers from back to front over your shoulder for a total of nine times on each shoulder.

2. At the highest point on the shoulder muscles, approximately half of the distance from the spine to the outer edge of the shoulder, is the pressure point called the *Shoulder Well*. Press firmly on this point with your middle finger for 30 seconds while you breathe deeply using the post-birth method. This *Shoulder Well* is a particularly effective point to relieve feelings of frustration and irritability.

3. On the same side, run your fingertips along the outside of your arm, over the middle finger, and to the juncture point on your palm where you should pause and press for a moment. To find this point, curl your fingers into a fist. Where the middle finger meets the palm is the *laogong* or junction of the two pathways that bring energy into your arms.

4. Then, continue using your fingertips from the juncture point back up the inside of your arm to your shoulder. Repeat nine times and then change sides.

5. Cross your arms and find the end of the elbow crease on the top of each arm. This point is called the *Crooked Pond*. Use this point to stimulate your immune system. It is also effective for relieving constipation, the fever of a cold, and arthritic pain in the elbow.

6. Press with your index or middle finger on the opposite elbow and hold for at least 30 seconds. Breathe deeply, using the post-birth method, while you press on these two acupressure points.

7. Now, press the flap of skin between your index finger and your thumb just in front of the joint between the two fingers with the thumb of your opposite hand. This is the *Joining the Valley* pressure point and is

helpful for increasing your immunity, cleansing your liver, or reducing feelings of depression. Hold for 30 seconds and then change hands.

8. Use a washing motion to massage the backs, palms, and fingers of your hands. Continue for a few seconds until your hands feel warm.

9. Using the opposite hand, press the blood from the base of each finger to the fingertip by massaging upward. Use a snapping motion at the tip of each finger to complete the massage.

10. Turn your wrist (either arm) so that the inside of the wrist is facing you. Run your finger along the wrist crease until you come to the end of it at the base of the little finger. This is the location of the *Spirit Gate*. Use this point to relieve anxiety and insomnia. Press and hold for 30 seconds as you breathe deeply.

11. Play the vertical flute by placing your left hand at the level of your abdomen and your right hand directly above it. Beginning with the little finger of your left hand, separate each finger, curling and uncurling as though you were pressing on the openings on the flute.

12. When you reach the top finger, which will be the thumb of your right hand, reverse the motion moving back down the imaginary flute. Repeat three times.

13. Change hands so that the right is now on the bottom and the left on top. Repeat the curling and uncurling of your fingers from hand to hand and back again. Again, do three runs up and down your imaginary flute.

Meditative relaxation

Benefits: The following mental exercises will relax the body, clear the mind, and restore the spirit to a state of balance and calm.

Posture: Check your patients' posture to make sure their backs are against the back of their chairs, feet are flat on the floor, toes turned slightly inward, and their legs are shoulder-width apart. Make sure they are sitting straight so that their heads are lightly suspended on their necks and their shoulders are rounded slightly forward but not hunched.

Point of origin: Direct your patients to bring their *qi* or energy upward from their lower *dan tians*. Remind them to move the energy with their minds through the middle *dan tian* that regulates the emotions and then to the upper *dan tian* that controls the mind and spirit.

Visualization for your patients: Imagine yourself floating on a cloud. Soothing, revitalizing energy passes from the top of your head, through your arms and trunk, and, finally, into your legs from where the *qi* flows back into the earth.

1. Close your eyes. Take a deep breath, expanding your diaphragm. Picture a flow of energy traveling up to the top of your head. Now, allow the energy to stream downward, flooding your head, neck, and face. Breathe out, gently contracting your diaphragm. Take two more deep, gentle breaths as you continue to visualize the energy flowing in and around your head and neck.

2. Now, mentally push the energy from your neck down into your shoulders, arms, and hands while you breathe deeply in and out for a total of three cleansing breaths.

3. From the shoulders, push the energy into your trunk, allowing the healing energy to circle in and around your organs and to travel up and down your spine. Take three long breaths while you envision the movement of the *qi*.

4. Direct the flow of energy from your trunk down into your hips, thighs, and knees. Allow the energy to circulate, soothing and relaxing overworked muscles and joints. Time the flow of the energy by taking three deep breaths in and out, using the post-birth method.

5. Then, direct the *qi* that you have released with your thoughts and, breathing deeply, send it into the lowest part of your legs, the calves, ankles, and, finally, the feet. We all exchange energy with our environment without realizing that the exchange is happening. Electromagnetic energy rises from the earth and is absorbed into the body through the soles of the feet. The energy or *qi* coursing through our bodies is returned to the earth as well, as it moves through our upper bodies, down our legs, and out through the soles of our feet.

ACUPRESSURE POINTS FOR RELAXATION

Stomach Meridian No. 3—Facial Beauty

Help your patients find this point by directing them to place their fingers at the bottom of their cheekbones directly below the pupils of their eyes. Have them press firmly and hold for at least 30 seconds.

Benefits: This point stimulates facial circulation, thereby improving the complexion. It may also be used to relieve acne and sinus congestion.

Stomach Meridian No. 2—Four Whites

Direct your patients to measure one finger-width below the lower ridge of the eye socket in line with the center of the iris. They will feel a slight indentation in the bone. Make sure they press on this pressure point firmly for one minute.

Benefits: This point is effective for relieving eye fatigue and pressure as well as headaches caused by stress.

Bladder Meridian No. 10—Heavenly Pillar

Help your patients find the two ropy muscles at the back of their necks. Ask them to measure or estimate approximately one half inch (1.25cm) below the base of the skull and press firmly for a full minute.

Benefits: This is a particularly potent point to alleviate stress, exhaustion, eyestrain, and feelings of burnout.

Stomach Meridian No. 6—Jaw Chariot

Ask your patients to clench their teeth until they feel the masseter muscle bulge between the upper and lower jaw. Have them press firmly on a point about midway between the upper and lower jaw for at least 30 seconds.

Benefits: Recommend to your patients that they use this point if they feel tension in their jaws or experience spasms in the jaw. This point may also be used for a sore throat or a toothache.

Triple Warmer Meridian No. 15—Heavenly Rejuvenation

Midway between the base of the neck and the outside edge of the shoulder at approximately one half inch (1.25cm) to the back of the shoulder muscle is the pressure point *Heavenly Rejuvenation*. Direct your patients to press firmly with the middle finger of their opposite hand for at least 30 seconds as they breathe deeply.

Benefits: Much of our stress is experienced as tension in the shoulders and stiffness in the neck. Recommend the use of this point to your patients whenever they begin to feel pain or stiffness in these areas.

Triple Warmer Meridian No. 4—Active Pond

Approximately half a thumb-width in from the outside of the arm on the crease below the wrist is the pressure point called *Active Pond*. Suggest that your patients press gently but steadily on this point for 30 seconds for arm and finger pain.

Benefits: Your patients may want to use this point often to relieve tension in their fingers and arms caused by repetitious motion.

Pericardium Meridian No. 7—Big Mound

This pressure point is located on the inside of the arm in the middle of the wrist crease. To help your patients relieve pain in their wrists, suggest that they press gently on this acupressure point for several seconds as they breathe deeply and concentrate on relaxing each muscle of their wrist.

Benefits: Like the pressure point described above (*Active Pond*), this point is beneficial for relieving the tension and pain of repetitive movements.

Pericardium Meridian No. 6—Inner Gate

Once again, this pressure point is on the inside of the forearm. To help your patients locate this point, ask them to measure two and one-half finger-widths below the wrist crease in the middle of their forearms. They should press gently on this point while taking several deep breaths and deliberately clearing their minds.

Benefits: This is an effective point for the relief of nausea and anxiety caused by stressful situations.

Option two

Exercises	Acupressure points
Head, Neck, and Shoulders	Conception Vessel No. 17—Sea of Tranquility
Trunk Rotations	Gall Bladder Meridian No. 21—Shoulder Well
Yoga Facelift	Heart Meridian No. 7—Spirit Gate
Centering Qi	Triple Warmer Meridian No. 16—Window of Heaven
Self-massage	Governing Vessel No. 19—Posterior Summit
Massage of abdomen, hips, and lower back	
Massage of legs and knees	
Meditative relaxation	

All breathing in this section of exercises, with the exception of *Centering Qi* is post-birth breathing—that is, the diaphragm is expanded when breathing in and contracted when breathing out.

HEAD, NECK, AND SHOULDERS

Benefits: This exercise will relax the muscles of the neck and realign the cervical vertebrae.

Posture: Check on your patients to make sure they are still sitting with their backs against the back of their chairs. Their legs should be shoulder-width apart, feet flat on the floor. Remind them to tuck their hips under slightly and curve their shoulders inward without hunching. The idea here is to keep the *qi* from flowing outward and away from the body. They should be holding their heads lightly on their necks as though their heads were suspended by a string from the ceiling.

Point of origin: Inform your patients that, in this exercise, the energy is released from the lower *dan tian* and spreads throughout their torsos as it passes through their middle and upper *dan tians*.

Visualization for your patients: Imagine that your head is a light ball perched on a flexible stalk and that your neck muscles are as elastic as an infant's.

1. Take a deep breath while your head is upright and then lower your head gently to your chest while you breathe out. Return your head

to the center as you breathe in. Lower your head backwards without straining as you breathe out. Counting the backward and forward motion as one, repeat nine times.

2. Breathe in deeply while your head is upright then let your head drop toward your right shoulder as you breathe out. Return your head to center and take a deep breath in again (using the post-birth breathing method) and let your head drop gently toward your left shoulder, breathing out as you do so. The side-to-side movements should be counted as one. Repeat the sequence for a total of nine times.

3. You will finish with your head over your right shoulder. Now, circle your head down to your chest and around to the left, then return to the center. Do not lean your head backward while circling. Circle your head nine times.

4. Begin with your head upright and then drop it gently toward your left shoulder, then right and so on for a total of nine times. Remember to breathe in deeply as you lift your head to the upright position. Continue alternating sides for a total of nine times.

5. On the ninth count, your head will be over your left shoulder. Circle your head down to your chest and then up to the right. Complete nine circles.

6. Finish in the upright position and then turn your head so that you are looking over your right shoulder. Come back to the center and look over your left shoulder. Each direction is counted as one.

7. When you finish, you will be looking over your right shoulder. Now, turn your head to the left, tilted upwards and looking toward the point where the wall and ceiling meet. Reverse and repeat, counting each side as one until you have completed nine turn and lift movements.

8. Now, shrug your shoulders lifting them up as close to your ears as possible. Allow them to drop abruptly. Continue lifting and dropping your shoulders for a total of nine times.

9. Circle your shoulders to the back nine times. Then, circle your shoulders forward nine times. Remember to do this gently without strain and to allow your arms to dangle loosely by your sides.

TRUNK ROTATIONS

Benefits: This exercise will loosen and stretch the muscles of your patients' backs and waists. In the process they will be reducing their waistlines and tightening their abdominal muscles.

Posture: Make sure your patients are sitting in the same position as in the previous exercises.

Point of origin: The *qi* is brought from the lower *dan tian* through the middle *dan tian*. As your patients bend over their thighs and release their breath, toxins are expelled from their lungs. As they return to an upright position, ask them to breathe in. That action will allow them to lift the *qi* all the way to the upper *dan tian*.

Visualization for your patients: Think about the energy being generated throughout your upper body. Imagine the destruction of fat particles as they are broken up and flushed through your system. All of the upper body is invigorated as energy passes through the meridians at the front, back, center, and waist. Juncture points are opened to release obstructions.

1. Begin again with your hands resting on your thighs.

2. Breathe in deeply, expanding your diaphragm.

3. Circle your trunk to the left, brushing the tops of your thighs with your chest (see Figure 3.13, page 127). Blow out your breath and tighten your abdomen.

4. Continue circling to the left side, and returning to the center.

5. Take a deep breath again and this time circle counterclockwise, blowing out your breath as you bend over your thighs.

6. From the center, circle your trunk to the right or counterclockwise, breathing in before you begin. Exhale as you reach the lowest point of the arc. Then, tighten your abdomen as your chest brushes the tops of your thighs.

7. Repeat nine times in each direction for a total of 18 repetitions.

YOGA FACELIFT

Benefits: This exercise increases circulation to the face and head. The result is a clearer mind, improved skin tone, and the reduction of fine lines and wrinkles.

Posture: Make sure your patients are seated in the same posture as in the previous exercise.

Point of origin: Energy rises from the lower *dan tian* in this exercise, passes through the middle *dan tian,* and fully envelops the upper *dan tian,* clearing the mind and sharpening the memory.

Visualization for your patients: Picture reversing the effect of the pull of gravity on your facial muscles. Imagine the increased flow of blood and energy to your brain.

1. Bend over from the hips so that your head is hanging down between your knees.

2. Allow your arms to dangle alongside your thighs.

3. Relax all the muscles of your face, lips slightly parted. You will be unable to breathe deeply during this time because your chest is resting on your thighs, so breathe lightly through your nose only.

4. Remain in this position for one minute if you are able to without becoming lightheaded or dizzy. If the position bothers you, reduce the time to 30 seconds and increase that time gradually as you become more comfortable in this position.

5. Regardless of the amount of time you spend in this position, breathe in as you return to your original posture by rolling upward until your back is straight and against the back of the chair once more. Use your abdominal muscles to pull yourself upright.

CENTERING QI

Benefits: This exercise will recenter the energy and rebalance your body.

Posture: Have your patients sit in the same posture as in the previous exercise.

Point of origin: Energy rises from the lower *dan tian,* circulates throughout the entire body, returning at last to the three repositories or *dan tians.*

Visualization for your patients: Imagine that you are collecting the *qi* and bits of energy from all over your body, returning them to a neutral position so that none will be lost or trapped elsewhere.

In this exercise, the pre-birth breathing method is used—that is, as you breathe in through your nose, contract your diaphragm, and as you breathe out, expand just your lower abdomen.

1. Hold your hands palm up just above your lap, fingertips touching (see Figure 2.2, page 27). Breathe in deeply through your nose while contracting your diaphragm. It is only in this one exercise that the diaphragm is *not* expanded during inhalations.

2. As you tighten your diaphragm and abdomen, raise your arms out to the side and up over your head to its center. Your palms are now facing the ceiling, fingers barely touching (see Figure 2.3, page 28).

3. Allow your arms to descend gradually in an arc out to the side. As you do so, exhale until there is no breath left in your lungs and relax just the muscles of your lower abdomen.

4. Return your arms to the original position in front of the lowest part of your abdomen, palms upward.

Self-massage

Massage of abdomen, hips, and lower back

Benefits: The brushing movements over the abdomen will firm the stomach while relieving bloating, constipation, and diarrhea. The circular motion of your patients' hands on their hips will warm the joints by increasing circulation to the area. The warmth of their hands combined with a firm pressure will alleviate the tension that accumulates in the lower back.

Posture: Have your patients remain seated in the same starting position as in the previous exercises.

Point of origin: Because they are concentrating this massage in the lower trunk and hip area, your patients will notice that the focus of the *qi* will remain around the lower *dan tian*.

Visualization for your patients: Imagine the energy passing around and through the intestines, circling around your hip joints, and sending waves of soothing energy through your lower back.

1. Hold one hand over the other at waist level. Brush downward with a firm pressure to about three finger-widths below the navel. Continue the brushing motion for about 30 seconds.

2. Measure two finger-widths directly below your navel. This is the location of the *Sea of Energy* pressure point. Press firmly on this point and hold for 30 seconds. (The *Sea of Energy* is an effective acupressure point for strengthening the abdominal and back muscles and for alleviating lower back pain.)

3. Now, move your hands to your right hip. Massage your hip using a circular motion around your hip from back to front. Change sides and repeat the circular motion. Press firmly to stimulate the circulation.

4. Sit forward in your chair. Place both hands on your lower back. Run your fingertips up and down your lower back. If you have a backache, circle your hands using the heels of your palms for a deeper massage.

5. Two finger-widths from your spine on either side between the second and third lumbar vertebrae is the pressure point B23, which is one of the *Sea of Vitality* points. B47, the second *Sea of Vitality* point, is four finger-widths from the spine (on either side) between the second and third lumbar vertebrae. Both of these points are awkward spots to reach and to press with just your fingers. Locate one set of the points first and then fist your hands at these spots and lean back against the back of your chair. This will ensure greater pressure and therefore quicker relief from pain and discomfort in your lower back.

6. Find the large bony area at the base of your spine. Measure two finger-widths from the spine to find the *Womb and Vitals* acupressure point. Again, these points are in an awkward place, so fisting your hands and leaning back against your chair will be of more benefit to you if you have a backache. Continue leaning back against your fists for at least 30 seconds.

Massage of legs and knees

Benefits: Use this massage and pressure point method for your patients who need to increase the circulation to their legs and relieve muscle aches. When they massage around their kneecaps, they will be promoting the production of synovial fluid for increased flexibility. The acupressure point on the outside of the leg benefits digestion and reduces fatigue. The pressure point at the back of the knee strengthens the lower back and the knees.

Posture: Make sure your patients begin in the usual position on their chairs. They will, of course, have to lean over to massage their legs and to use the acupressure points in this section. Let them know that they will not be able to breathe as deeply nor expand their diaphragms as much when they are bent over. Therefore, when they have completed each part of the massage, instruct your patients to return to an upright position and take two or three deep, cleansing breaths.

Point of origin: Again, you and your patients will be targeting the lower *dan tian* during these exercises. Remember to direct them to use their minds to move the energy into the areas they are massaging.

Visualization for your patients: Picture the increased flow of blood and energy through your legs and around your knees.

1. Using the fingertips of your right hand, follow the meridian on the outside of your right leg to the top of your foot. Using both hands, circle your ankle joint. Then, run your fingertips up the inside of your leg to just below the top of your thigh. Repeat at least nine times.

2. Reverse hands and massage down your left leg to the foot and around your ankle. Bring the energy back up your leg to just below the top of your thigh. Again, repeat nine or more times.

3. Now, measure four finger-widths below your knee on the outside of the leg where there is a good-size indentation. This pressure point is called the *Three Mile Point*. This is a particularly effective point for the relief of bloating, cramps, nausea, and indigestion. Press firmly with your middle fingers (one on each leg) and hold for 30 seconds.

4. Move your hands to the back of your legs and press both thumbs in the middle of the creases at the back of your knees. This is the location of the acupressure point called the *Commanding Middle*. If you suffer from backache, knee pain or stiffness, arthritis of the knee, or sciatica, this is a pressure point you will want to use regularly. Press strongly on these two points and hold for at least 30 seconds.

5. Next to the bone on the inside of your ankle is a small indentation. This is the pressure point called *Joyful Sleep*. It is, as the name implies, an effective point to relieve insomnia. Press firmly on this point for at least 30 seconds, preferably just before bedtime, to ensure a good night's sleep.

6. On the outside of your ankle near the bottom of the large ankle bone is another small hollow. This is the *Calm Sleep* acupressure point. Press firmly on this point with your middle finger and hold for 30 seconds. This is another point that may be used before going to bed at night or to create a feeling of calm at any time during the day.

MEDITATIVE RELAXATION

Benefits: The following exercise will help your patients clear their minds, relax their bodies, and restore their spirits so that they will feel calm and centered.

Posture: Check your patients' posture to make certain their feet are flat on the floor, toes turned slightly inward. Their legs should be approximately shoulder-width apart and their backs must be flat against the chair so that they cannot slide their hands between their backs and the back of the chair. Remind them to round their shoulders forward slightly, allowing their hands to rest comfortably on their thighs.

Point of origin: Once again, your patients will be moving the energy (with their breath and their minds) from the lower *dan tian* up and through the middle and upper *dan tians* as the *qi* circulates throughout the entire body.

Visualization for your patients: Put yourself in a relaxed mood and concentrate on the directions.

1. Take several deep and cleansing breaths—in through your nose, expanding your diaphragm, and out through your mouth, contracting your diaphragm.

2. Imagine that you are in a hot air balloon. Think about the color and design of the envelope. Visualize the shape and color of the basket.

3. Now, breathing in and out through your nose only, begin your imaginary trip. You are safely tucked in the basket. The colorful envelope is holding you aloft as you sail through the clear blue sky with only birds for company. As you float far above the earth, continue to breathe in and out through your nose, allowing your diaphragm to expand as you breathe in and contract as you blow out.

ACUPRESSURE POINTS FOR RELAXATION

Conception Vessel Meridian No. 17—Sea of Tranquility

The *Sea of Tranquility* is located on the center of the breastbone, three finger-widths from its base. Direct your patients to press gently but firmly on this point for 30 seconds.

Benefits: Use this point for patients whenever they seem to be feeling nervous, anxious, or depressed. This point may also be used for hysteria or any other emotional imbalance.

Gall Bladder Meridian No. 21—Shoulder Well

To help your patients locate this acupressure point, have them press firmly on the highest point of their shoulder muscles approximately one to two inches (2.5–5cm) from the side of the lower neck. Make sure they maintain pressure on this point for at least 30 seconds. If any of your patients are pregnant, they may use this point but must press very lightly for the minimum amount of time.

Benefits: This is an effective acupressure point to relieve anxiety, irritability, nervous problems, headaches, poor circulation, or cold hands or feet.

Heart Meridian No. 7—Spirit Gate

Instruct your patients to run a finger along the outside of their forearms to the crease at their wrists. Have them use their thumbs to press on this point for at least 30 seconds.

Benefits: When you have a patient who is feeling anxious or nervous or experiencing periods of forgetfulness, suggest that they use this point for relief.

Triple Warmer Meridian No. 16—Window of Heaven

Help your patients locate this point by directing them to trace a line from the back of their earlobes to the first large indentation at the base of the skull. Make sure they press strongly with their index or middle fingers for at least 30 seconds.

Benefits: You may wish to recommend the use of this point for your patients to relieve their shoulder tension, neck pain, or headaches caused by stress.

Governing Vessel Meridian No. 19—Posterior Summit

So that your patients can find this point, have them run their fingers up the back of their heads to the top of their heads. Now, they should slide their fingers down the back of their heads a short distance until they can feel an indentation. Ask them to press firmly on this point with their middle fingers for 30 to 60 seconds.

Benefits: The *Posterior Summit* is a potent pressure point to alleviate feelings of depression, vertigo, or headaches. This acupressure point is also a good one to help your patients improve their memories.

Option three

Exercises	Acupressure points
An	Governing Vessel No. 21—Anterior Summit
Push Up Sky/Press Down on Earth	Pericardium Meridian No. 7—Big Mound
Hands Waving in Clouds	Conception Vessel No. 12—Center of Power
Centering Qi	Pericardium Meridian No. 3—Crooked Marsh
Self-massage	Lung Meridian No. 10—Fish Border
Massage of shoulder and arms	
Massage of abdomen, hips, and lower back	
Massage of legs and knees	
Meditative relaxation	

All breathing in this section of exercises, with the exception of *Centering Qi*, is post-birth breathing—that is, the diaphragm is expanded when breathing in and contracted when breathing out.

AN

Benefits: This exercise will massage and stimulate your patients' internal organs while stretching the muscles of their shoulders and arms.

Posture: Make sure your patients begin by sitting with their backs against the back of the chair. Their legs should be shoulder-width apart, feet flat on the floor. Remind them to tuck their hips under slightly and curve their shoulders inward without hunching. The idea here is to keep the *qi* from flowing outward and away from the body. They should hold their heads lightly on their necks as though their heads were suspended by a string from the ceiling.

Point of origin: You will be helping your patients to bring the energy upward from the lower *dan tian*. They should allow the *qi* to flow through their trunks and rise upward through their shoulders, necks, and heads.

Visualization for your patients: Think of your hands pressing against the molecules of air as you exchange energy with your immediate surroundings.

1. Hold your hands, palms forward, in front of your shoulders. Twist to your left and push your arms out to the side until your elbows are nearly straight (see Figure 3.3, page 94).

2. Bring your arms back in front of your shoulders, breathe in, twist to your right, and push your arms out as you exhale.

3. Continue alternating sides for a total of 18 pushes.

PUSH UP SKY/PRESS DOWN ON EARTH

Benefits: This exercise will stretch your patients' arm muscles while their waistlines are reduced and their abdominal muscles are tightened and strengthened.

Posture: Check to be sure your patients are still seated in the same position as that described in the previous exercise.

Point of origin: The movement of energy begins in the lower *dan tian* and travels throughout the body.

Visualization for your patients: Imagine that you are creating a space between the sky and the earth, and by touching each you are connecting with the energies of both.

1. Begin with your hands resting on your thighs.

2. Bring your right arm up, palm facing the ceiling, and at the same time press downward with your left hand, palm facing the floor (see Figure 3.1, page 86). Breathe in through your nose and expand your diaphragm.

3. Bring both arms, elbows bent, to the level of your solar plexus. Breathe out through your mouth. Tighten your diaphragm and abdomen and hold until you need to breathe in again.

4. Reverse your hands so that the left one reaches toward the ceiling this time and the right is pressing downward. Continue alternating sides, breathing in deeply as one arm ascends and the other descends, for a total of 18 repetitions.

HANDS WAVING IN CLOUDS

Benefits: The following exercise will strengthen your patients' shoulder and upper arm muscles while trimming their waistlines.

Posture: Check to be sure your patients are sitting in the same position as in the previous exercise.

Point of origin: Instruct your patients to bring the energy upward from the lower *dan tian* and push it upward through their middle and upper *dan tians*.

Visualization for your patients: Imagine that you are brushing wisps of clouds from in front of your face, chest, and abdomen.

1. Begin with your left hand at eye level and your right hand directly in front of the lower *dan tian* at the lowest part of your abdomen (see Figure 3.4, page 95).

2. Twist from your waist to the left, left hand held horizontally in front of your face. Leading with the inside of your wrist, allow your right hand to travel with the movement of your trunk as you twist to the left. Fingers should not be stiff and should be held apart so that you can look between your fingers. By allowing the muscles around your waist to relax and by breathing out as you twist, you will be able to turn much further to the side.

3. Sweep back and forth as your twist from side to side, changing which hand is on top each time. Continue the sweeps nine times on each side for a total of 18 waves. Most importantly, remember that the movement is gentle and loose, arms sweeping gracefully from side to side.

CENTERING QI

Benefits: This exercise will recenter the energy and rebalance the body.

Posture: Remind your patients to remain seated in the same posture as in the previous exercise.

Point of origin: Energy rises from the lower *dan tian,* circulates throughout the entire body, returning at last to the three repositories or *dan tians.*

Visualization for your patients: Imagine that you are collecting the *qi* and bits of energy from all over your body, returning them to a neutral position so that none will be lost or trapped elsewhere.

In this exercise, the pre-birth breathing method is used—that is, as you breathe in through your nose, contract your diaphragm, and as you breathe out, expand just your lower abdomen.

1. Hold your hands palm up just above your lap, fingertips touching (see Figure 2.2, page 27). Breathe in deeply through your nose while contracting your diaphragm. It is only in this one exercise that the diaphragm is *not* expanded during inhalations.

2. As you tighten your diaphragm and abdomen, raise your arms out to the side and up over your head to its center. Your palms are now facing the ceiling, fingers barely touching (see Figure 2.3, page 28).

3. Allow your arms to descend gradually in an arc out to the side. As you do so, exhale until there is no breath left in your lungs and relax just the muscles of your lower abdomen.

4. Return your arms to the original position in front of the lowest part of your abdomen, palms upward.

SELF-MASSAGE

Massage of shoulders and arms

Benefits: The self-massage and use of acupressure points will relax your patients' shoulders and arms if their muscles have become tense or strained during the previous exercises.

Posture: Instruct your patients to remain seated in the same position as in the previous exercises.

Point of origin: While the energy originates in the lower *dan tian,* much of the action of the *qi* will be in the middle *dan tian.*

Visualization for your patients: Imagine the soothing warmth of the energy as it moves through your shoulders and up and down the meridians of your arms. With your opposite hand, brush your fingers from back to front over your shoulder for a total of nine times on each shoulder.

1. At the highest point on the shoulder muscle, approximately half of the distance from the spine to the outer edge of the shoulder, is the pressure point called the *Shoulder Well.* Press firmly on this point with your middle finger for 30 seconds while you breathe deeply using the post-birth method. This *Shoulder Well* is a particularly effective point to relieve feelings of frustration and irritability.

2. On the same side, run your fingertips along the outside of your arm, over the middle finger, and to the juncture point on your palm where you should pause and press for a moment. To find this point, curl your fingers into a fist. Where the middle finger meets the palm is the *laogong* or junction of the two pathways that bring energy into your arms.

3. Then, continue using your fingertips from the juncture point back up the inside of your arm to your shoulder. Repeat nine times and then change sides.

4. Cross your arms and find the end of the elbow crease on the top of each arm. This point is called the *Crooked Pond.* Use this point to stimulate your immune system. It is also effective for relieving constipation, the fever of a cold, and arthritic pain in the elbow.

5. Press with your index or middle finger on the opposite elbow and hold for at least 30 seconds. Breathe deeply using the post-birth method while you press on these two acupressure points.

6. Now, press the flap of skin between your index finger and your thumb just in front of the joint between the two fingers with the thumb of your opposite hand. This is the *Joining the Valley* pressure point and is helpful for increasing your immunity, cleansing your liver, or reducing feelings of exhaustion and depression. Hold for 30 seconds and then change hands.

7. Use a washing motion to massage the backs, palms, and fingers of your hands. Continue for a few seconds until your hands feel warm.

8. Using the opposite hand, press the blood from the base of each finger to the fingertip by massaging upward. Use a snapping motion at the tip of each finger to complete the massage.

9. Turn your wrist (either arm) so that the inside of the wrist is facing you. Run your finger along the wrist crease until you come to the end of it at the base of the little finger. This is the location of the *Spirit Gate*. Use this point to relieve anxiety and insomnia caused by fatigue. Press and hold for 30 seconds as you breathe deeply.

10. Play an imaginary vertical flute by placing your left hand at the level of your abdomen and your right hand directly above it. Beginning with the little finger of your left hand, separate each finger, curling and uncurling as though you were pressing on the openings on the flute.

11. When you reach the top finger, which will be the thumb of your right hand, reverse the motion moving back down the imaginary flute. Repeat three times.

12. Change hands so that the right is now on the bottom and the left on top. Repeat the curling and uncurling of the fingers from hand to hand and back again. Again, make three runs up and down the flute.

Massage of abdomen, hips, and lower back

Benefits: The brushing movement of your patients' hands will soothe and tighten the abdominal muscles for a firmer, flatter stomach. At the same time, the downward motion of the massage can eliminate bloating and relieve either constipation or diarrhea. Direct your patients to use a circular motion for their hips to warm their joints by increasing the circulation to that area. At any time the muscles of the lower back are tense or painful, remind your patients to follow the steps in this exercise for relaxing their muscles and to relieve discomfort.

Posture: Remind your patients to begin seated in the same position as in the previous exercises. Check their postures periodically to make certain that your patients are seated with their backs against the back of their chairs and their legs are shoulder-width apart.

Point of origin: Since the massaging motions are concentrated in the lower abdomen, hip, and back area, energy from the lower *dan tian* is being directly stimulated.

Visualization for your patients: Imagine energy passing around and through the intestines, circling around the hip joints, and sending waves of soothing *qi* through the lower back.

1. Hold one hand over the other at waist level. Brush downward with gentle but firm pressure to about three finger-widths below your navel. Continue the brushing movement for about 30 seconds.

2. Measure two finger-widths below your navel to the pressure point called *Gate Origin*. Press firmly and hold for at least 30 seconds. Use this point to tone weak abdominal muscles, strengthen your back, and alleviate back pain.

3. Using both hands, alternately press and massage around your hips in a circular motion. Continue massaging for 30 seconds and then change to the other hip.

4. Now, sit forward on your chair and place both hands on your lower back. Run your fingertips up and down your back with a firm pressure. If you have pain in your back, circle your hands using the heels of your palms for a deeper massage.

5. B23 and B47 (the two *Sea of Vitality* points) are in line with each other on your back between the second and third lumbar vertebrae. B23 is two finger-widths from your spine on either side. B47 is four finger-widths from the spine on either side. Because these may be awkward spots to reach, locate the areas with your fingers then fist your hands at those spots and lean back against the back of your chair. Continue to lean back against your fists as they are pressed on these two spots for at least 30 to 60 seconds.

6. Find the large bony area at the base of your spine. Measure one to two finger-widths from the spine to find the *Womb and Vitals* acupressure points. Because of the location of these points, fist your hands again and lean back into the back of your chair. Breathe deeply and hold for 30 seconds.

Massage of legs and knees

Benefits: The motion of your patients' hands will stimulate the circulation in their legs, relieving muscle aches. Massaging around the kneecaps will promote the production of synovial fluid for increased flexibility. The acupressure point on the outside of the leg benefits digestion and reduces fatigue, while the point at the back of the knee strengthens the lower back and knees.

Posture: Make sure your patients begin in the seated position they were in during the previous exercise.

Point of origin: Let your patients know that energy will be released from the lower *dan tian* as they massage their legs and knees.

Visualization for your patients: Breathing deeply, direct the movement of the energy with your mind as you picture the *qi* traveling to the areas you are massaging.

1. Using the fingertips of your right hand, follow the meridian on the outside of your right leg to the top of your foot. Using both hands, circle your ankle joint. Then, run the fingertips of your left hand up the inside of your leg to just below the top of your thigh. Continue for at least nine times before changing to your right leg.

2. Now, measure four finger-widths below your knee on the outside of each leg. Find the large depression and press with your middle fingers firmly on this point for at least 30 seconds. This is the *Three Mile Point* and is particularly effective for the relief of bloating, cramps, nausea, and indigestion.

3. Take a deep breath in through your nose. Lean forward and press both thumbs at the point called the *Commanding Middle* which, as the name implies, is located in the middle of the creases in the back of your knees. If you suffer from backaches, knee pain or stiffness, arthritis of the knee, or sciatica, this is a pressure point you will want to use regularly. Breathe out slowly through your mouth and hold for the full length of the breath. Release and then breathe in deeply again and press firmly on these acupressure points.

4. Trace your finger to the bone on the inside of your ankle. There is a small indentation next to the bone. This pressure point is called *Joyful Sleep*. As its name implies, it is an effective point to relieve insomnia. Press firmly on this point and hold for at least 30 seconds. Using this point at bedtime will ensure a good night's sleep.

5. There is another pressure point that is helpful at bedtime. *Calm Sleep* is beneficial for relieving chronic back pain. To locate this point, slide your finger down the large ankle bone on the outside of your leg until you find the first, small indentation. Take a deep breath as you press firmly on this point. Release your breath through your mouth slowly.

Continue breathing in and out and hold your finger at the point of *Calm Sleep* for about 30 seconds while concentrating on the movement of energy to your lower back.

MEDITATIVE RELAXATION

Benefits: The following mental exercises will relax your patients' bodies, clear their minds, and restore their spirits to a state of balance and calm.

Posture: Check your patients' postures to make sure their backs are against the back of their chairs, their feet are flat on the floor, toes turned slightly inward, and their legs are shoulder-width apart. Make sure they are sitting straight so that their heads are lightly suspended on their necks and their shoulders are rounded slightly forward but not hunched.

Point of origin: This exercise will bring the *qi* or energy upward from the lower *dan tian*. Remind your patients that they are moving the energy with their minds through the middle *dan tian* that regulates the emotions, then to the upper *dan tian* which controls your mind and spirit.

Visualization for your patients: Imagine yourself floating on a cloud. Soothing energy passes from the top of your head, through your arms and trunk, and finally into your legs from where the *qi* flows back into the earth.

1. Close your eyes. Take a deep breath, expanding your diaphragm. Picture a flow of energy traveling up to the top of your head. Now, allow the energy to stream downward flooding your head, neck, and face. Breathe out gently, contracting your diaphragm. Take two more deep, gentle breaths as you continue to visualize the energy flowing in and around your head and neck.

2. Now, mentally push the energy from your neck down into your shoulders, arms, and hands while you breathe deeply in and out for a total of three cleansing breaths.

3. From the shoulders, push the energy into your trunk, allowing the healing energy to circle in and around your organs and to travel up and down your spine. Take three long breaths while you envision the movement of the *qi*.

4. Direct the flow of energy from your trunk down into your hips, thighs, and knees. Allow the energy to circulate, soothing and relaxing overworked muscles and joints. Time the flow of the energy by taking three deep breaths in and out, using the post-birth method.

5. Then, direct the *qi* that you have released with your thoughts and deep breathing into the lowest part of your legs, the calves, ankles, and finally the feet. We all exchange energy with our environment without realizing that the exchange is happening. Electromagnetic energy rises from the earth and is absorbed into the body through the soles of the feet. The energy or *qi* coursing through our bodies is returned to the earth as it moves through our upper bodies, down our legs, and out through the soles of our feet as well.

Acupressure points for relaxation

Governing Vessel Meridian No. 21—Anterior Summit

Help your patients find this pressure point by asking them to place their fingers behind their left and right ears. Direct them to move their fingertips in a straight line to slightly back of the top of their heads where there is a hollow. Now, have them move their fingertips to approximately one inch (2.5cm) in front of that hollow. They should press firmly at this location and hold for at least 30 seconds.

Benefits: Use this point for patients who complain of headaches, feelings of depression, and memory loss.

Pericardium Meridian No. 7—Big Mound

This pressure point can be found on the inside of the arm at the middle of the wrist crease. Direct your patients to press gently but firmly on this point for 30 to 60 seconds.

Benefits: If any of your patients are experiencing wrist pain or tendonitis from repetitious activity, suggest that they use this point often.

Conception Vessel Meridian No. 12—Center of Power

Ask your patients to measure three finger-widths below the base of their breastbones in the pit of the upper stomach. Make sure they press firmly but not too deeply and hold for at least two minutes. It is best for your patients to use this point when their stomachs are relatively empty.

Benefits: This point is effective for the relief of indigestion, heartburn, constipation, abdominal spasms, and emotional stress.

Pericardium Meridian No. 3—Crooked Marsh

Instruct your patients to bend their arms and with the opposite finger press on the lower end of the inside of the elbow. They should press on this point for at least 30 to 60 seconds.

Benefits: This is an effective acupressure point for your patients when they are experiencing a nervous stomachache or feelings of anxiety.

Lung Meridian No. 10—Fish Border

On the palm side of their hands, your patients will find the center of the pad at the base of the thumb. Have them press firmly and hold for a full minute.

Benefits: Suggest this point to your patients who need to alleviate lung problems such as coughing spells and asthma.

4

THE ROLE OF
STRESS IN DISEASE

If only stress could be seen, isolated, and measured, I am sure we could enormously lengthen the human life span.

Hans Selye, MD, PhD
Founder of the International Institute of Stress, Montreal, Canada

Dr. Selye and other practicing physicians and researchers define biological stress as a "nonspecific response within the body to any environmental demand." These researchers have concluded that 60 to 90 percent of all diseases are stress-related. Lack of sleep, poor diet, environmental toxins, and pressures at work and at home can be counted among the most common stressors. The predisposition to diabetes, for example, is thought to be inherited. We know that diet plays an important role as well. However, many researchers now believe that the level of development of the disease is the result of the level of stress experienced by that person and the way in which he/she reacts to that stress. After many years of research with diabetic patients, Dr. Selye concluded that genetic predisposition and an insufficiency of insulin formation are not the only contributing factors. He discovered that these patients excreted unusually high amounts of peptic digestive hormones in their urine, which led him to theorize that two additional agents might be contributing to the development of the disease. He believed that the combination of stress and anti-inflammatory hormonal treatments would result in the over-production of such adaptive (protein) hormones as ACTH, STH, or COL, and would produce a spike in the blood sugar levels of these patients. The already weakened inflammatory barricades are then further compromised by a treatment that allows the "attacking influence" of the digestive juices to increase as the hormones stimulate more production of peptic enzymes. For a more in-depth study of this topic, see Selye (undated).

At the same time that neurologists and researchers began to discover the connection between stress and illness, the notion of mind–body medicine became more widely accepted. When we think of health, we tend to concentrate on diet and exercise as the solution to all ills. But recent studies have proven the link between a person's mental state and attitude and the ability to control and even cure certain diseases. In one such study, Parkinson's disease patients were told that they were to receive a new surgical procedure that would reduce the symptoms of their disease. These patients showed marked improvement after their experimental surgery even though the surgeons did no more than drill a small hole in their skulls and then patch it. PET scans after the sham surgery clearly showed a significant rise in dopamine in these patients that was equal to, if not greater than, that shown in other patients who received active treatment for their disease. In other words, the so-called "placebo response" was not an imaginary lessening of symptoms but a true, measurable change. In fact, researchers at UCLA have discovered that optimism produces a stronger than normal immune cell function and that certain exercises (even those as simple as deep breathing) can dramatically reduce chronic stress. In a relaxed state, the body produces more nitric oxide than usual and this molecule is believed to act as an antidote to cortisol and other toxic stress hormones. Dr. Herbert Benson, in the article in the September 27, 2004 issue of *Newsweek* from which the above information was taken, suggests that the brain may very well be a "gateway" to the tissue and organs of the human body. He states that the challenge now is to establish a map to the pathways that link mental states to measurable medical changes in the body. From there, doctors and researchers will be able to better assess medical problems and to find solutions to those problems.

It is my belief that this research was begun thousands of years ago and that those pathways have already been mapped by ancient Eastern medical practitioners, both in practice and in the medical texts that have survived through the centuries. How ironic it would be if we have had the solution to these problems all along!

Stress and your environment

Stress can have a positive effect on our lives or a negative one. Scientists believe that "stress" is the modern version of the "flight or fight" response essential to the survival of our early ancestors. Fear of realistic dangers prepared us to take defensive action to save ourselves from injury or even death. In moderate doses, stress may motivate us to do our best work, stimulate our creativity, or push us to complete a task in the most efficient manner possible.

On the negative side, stress may lead to psychological and/or physical ailments. Faced with a task that appears insurmountable, the memory of past failures and tension from a previous incident can resurface before work even begins. Eventually, just thinking about a similarly difficult or complex assignment can trigger all the symptoms we experienced in the previous situation. Repeated stress over an extended period of time creates a vicious cycle of anxiety leading to tension-building thoughts that bring on the symptoms of stress-induced physical illness. As the stressful situation continues, our "flight or fight" response spirals out of control. In a worst case scenario, the result may be the onset of a serious and prolonged illness.

Yet, stress is a part of everyday life and so is the fatigue that accompanies it. Because we cannot avoid it, we must be proactive in learning to deal with the pressures we face every day.

Since the purpose of this book is to present an exercise program that reduces the unhealthy effects of stress in your own and your patients' daily lives, it would not be off the subject to discuss the arrangement of your own personal environment and the area where you work with patients as an additional means to reduce stress and fatigue for you and for them.

For you to be successful in your practice of healing with Taiji and Qigong, you should be aware of the surroundings where you work with patients. Positive energy in your work area will allow both you and your patients to use the energy in the environment interactively with the internal energy that has been stimulated during the exercise session. When the energy in your home, office, or work area is negative, every activity you undertake in that place will also be negative. Clutter, misplaced files, or an inharmonious arrangement of your work or relaxation space can be at the root of feelings of helplessness and inadequacy when you are faced with a difficult case or an unpleasant situation with co-workers and can adversely affect your work with patients. In addition to the often recommended stress reducers such as exercise, meditation, and altering patterns of thought, the art of Feng Shui can serve as a guide to improving your immediate surroundings so that some common causes of stress for you and those you are working to heal are lessened.

Feng Shui

Like Taijiquan, Feng Shui is based on the five elements of wind, water, earth, metal, and fire, the Yi Jing, and the Taiji diagram. It is an environmental science whose purpose is to create a harmonious space for living and working.

The words themselves literally mean wind and water: wind provides the movement or flow of *qi*; the water is the container or receiver of the *qi*.

Feng Shui is sometimes referred to as the "art of balance." It is an ancient system for designing an individual room, the floor plan of a house, or the construction and furnishing of a large commercial building. Observation, reflection, and plain old common sense are essential to the successful application of the principles of Feng Shui to a room or a building. Feng Shui is fundamentally a right-brain activity based on intuition and feelings but directed or channeled through the use of certain instruments such as the *luo pan* and the *bagua*.

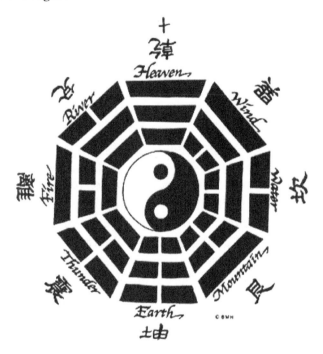

Figure 4.1 The bagua

A *luo pan* is a complex instrument dating back several thousand years. All versions of the *luo pan* contain many concentric rings. These rings represent such fundamentals as the 64 hexagrams of the Yi Jing, the five elements, and the directions of a compass. The *bagua* is a simplified version of the *luo pan* and, as such, is a more efficient and usable tool for those of us who are amateurs in the applications of Feng Shui. Each of the sides of the *bagua* represents a direction of the compass. Each direction relates to one of the five elements and one of four animals out of a total of 12 animals used in Chinese astrology.

As a first step, the *bagua* provides guidance in the placement of furniture and accessories that will lend a feeling of peace and contentment to any living or working space and colors appropriate to the purpose of the room or the nature of the business. For example, red represents fame and may be used in the corresponding area of a room or a house. The color green (wood) is ideal for new businesses because it represents new growth. Since brown is the color of the earth, various shades of brown, beige, and cream used as the predominant color scheme will lend a feeling of stability to a business that is volatile by its nature. For a newly created or re-created company, the color white represents a fresh start. If you are able to change the colors in your office, are starting a new business, or feel you need to have a new look in your home or work space, many fine books on the art of Feng Shui contain complete charts of appropriate colors for every situation. Some of these books are listed in the Bibliography (Appendix C) at the back of the book.

While the *bagua* is a less complex and more easily understood Feng Shui tool than the original *luo pan*, it too can be broken down further into a nine-section square. This square is often referred to as the "magic square." Each of the sections represents an aspect of our lives. That portion of our lives can be strengthened with the proper use of color, symbols, mirrors, and so on. Figure 4.2 shows each of those sections as they would be illustrated in a room or house that is perfectly square.

Wealth	Fame	Marriage
Family and Health	Good Luck Center	Children
Knowledge	Career	Mentors and Travel

Figure 4.2 Magic square

Keep in mind that a door is rarely located in the exact center of a room. Therefore, the entry to any room or to a home may be in the "Mentors and travel" or the "Knowledge" section of the area rather than in the "Career" section as would be the case if the doorway were directly centered in the "entry" wall. In such a situation, the *qi* is simply entering your room or your home through the "Mentors and travel" or "Knowledge" sections. This doesn't necessarily present a problem for you. In fact, these alternative entry sections may be advantageous, particularly if the door to your business, your office, or your therapy area is in the "Mentors and travel" area. Again, depending upon the nature of your particular business or hobby—for example, if you are involved in any of the arts such as writing, painting, sculpting, performing, or healing—entry of the *qi* through the intuitive area may be the best possible arrangement.

Cutouts that provide closet space or an extended area of an adjacent room may result in a missing portion of the room. Buildings are rarely perfectly rectangular or perfectly square. Often important sections may not be included in the design of a house or place of business. When you encounter such a situation, there are simple ways to return the area to a state of balance. If it is your home that is missing a vital area, such outdoor additions as plantings, paving stones, or birdbaths can replace the missing piece. In the case of a room that is lacking a vital area of your life as indicated on the magic square, the addition of plants, a tabletop waterfall, or a mirror may be the most effective and least expensive solution.

Whatever the case, George Birdsall, in his book *The Feng Shui Companion* (2007), recommends nine basic cures to increase the movement of *qi* in your home or office. The "nine basic cures" are mobiles, plants, wind chimes, windmills, bells, crystals, fountains, mirrors, music, and a fish bowl or aquarium. Use of any of these items in an area that requires strengthening should be based on your own personal preference and on how the addition of one or more of these items makes you "feel" about the room. A Feng Shui professional may recommend a particular cure, but the ultimate decision is up to you and your intuition. If you are more comfortable as a result of adding a wind chime, if you and your patients find the room more welcoming when it is enhanced by a lush, green plant or a colorful fish swimming around in a bowl, then that is the cure for you. In addition, there are certain other "rules of thumb" that apply to both your home and your place of business:

1. Use only rounded leaf plants, particularly in a relationship area. Spiky plants should be placed only in a location where protection is required such as the entry to a very private space.

2. Open beams can sometimes create negative *qi* with the feeling of something "hanging over your head." If at all possible, never place anything as important as a desk on which business is conducted, or your bed, under a beam.

3. Never place your desk so that your back is to the door. If there is not enough space to relocate your desk, hang a decorative but clear mirror over the desk so that you can see people as they enter your office.

4. No table, desk, or therapy bed should be in a direct line with the door. *Qi* should flow in a circular pattern, not in a straight line.

5. As a general rule, don't use mirror tiles or split mirrors since they have a tendency to "split" your image. Again, these items can produce negative *qi* because you and your patients may feel as though you're being pulled in different directions.

6. Use the magic square or a *bagua* and then place appropriate objects or objects with appropriate colors in those areas.

Clean up the clutter!

Clutter is the most common and most invasive hindrance to the free flow of *qi*. If you are a collector of old paint cans, remnants, buttons, or other miscellaneous odds and ends, change your ways. Think of the last time you moved or did your spring cleaning. Remember the feeling of release and lightness you experienced as a result of disposing of all those things you thought you couldn't live without?

Unfortunately, many of us are reluctant to throw anything away—just in case we might find a need for it later on. Clothes that have not been worn for two or three years should be discarded. Keeping old clothes that you will probably never wear again adds to the clutter in your home and impedes the proper flow of *qi*. If an item is not attractive, if you cannot find the proper spot for it, or, more importantly, if it has a negative memory attached to it, don't allow guilt to keep you from selling it or giving it away. Most Feng Shui experts agree that certain energies are attached to objects and that those objects may have an adverse affect on the overall *qi* in your home.

Clutter in offices is of a different sort. There is a sign that reads "A messy desk is a sign of genius." A genius perhaps, but that person will certainly not be productive. A desk piled high with papers and files is indicative of a cluttered mind, one that is unable to finish projects, prioritize their importance, or handle multiple tasks. In this day and age of "multitasking" and speed of communication, most employees as well as business owners are required to juggle several assignments at the same time, so it is doubly important to be well organized.

Fortunately, a wide range of desktop computers, laptops, tablets, smart phones, and various digital accessories can make our working lives easier. Many of these items are costly but may be worth the price if more work can be accomplished in a shorter span of time, thereby reducing your stress level. If your working area is small, cloud computing or a thumb drive can cut down on the paper and file clutter and free up a great deal of space.

There are disadvantages, of course, to relying completely on electronic gadgets—a high price tag, the time necessary to input all your information and to learn a new system, and the loss of important files if the system fails. If you are self-employed, the decision is ultimately yours. Buy only those items that you can afford and only those that will make you more productive. As in all other aspects of Feng Shui, common sense and intuition should be your guide when purchasing any new equipment. The following are a few basic rules to help you save time, eliminate frustrations, and accomplish more in a shorter amount of time, whether you are an employee of a large company or are self-employed:

1. Organize your work so that files are well marked whether in a filing cabinet or in folders on your computer.

2. Put your files in the order in which they will be used.

3. Clean out your "in" basket (emails, IMs (instant messages), etc.) as quickly as possible.

4. Don't handle the same piece of paper or the same digital file more than once.

Above all, your work space should be pleasant and welcoming. Mementos and photos will personalize a work space. Select the suitable colors and location for your personal items. Use the magic square for the proper placement of your furniture and replace "empty" sections with one or more of the nine basic cures. Live plants and a tabletop waterfall can turn even the most sterile office into an agreeable spot in which to work. A poster or painting of a pleasant scene—while not as good as a natural setting—can relieve the bleakness of bare walls. If you have a window and that window looks out onto a grassy area with trees and flowers, so much the better. Ultimately, what you choose to put in your office can make all the difference to how you feel each morning when you walk through the door. And, in the long run, you can reduce the level of stress in your life, avoid frustration and disease, and be a more effective healer.

Reducing fatigue and stress with water

Most of us have the habit of drinking coffee or sodas throughout the day. The caffeine in coffee and in most soft drinks actually depletes the body of the very fluid it needs. Worse yet, the caffeine may cause us to lose our ability to accurately determine our level of dehydration. We may mistake our decreased level of fluids as hunger or we may assume we are just tired. It is true that coffee and pop are made with water, but if they are caffeinated, the amount absorbed by the body is actually *decreased*. The more coffee or soda we drink, the more fluid we lose from our tissues. The caffeine in sodas, in coffee, and, less drastically, in tea acts as a diuretic, removing not excess fluid from the body but the water that is essential to good mental, physical, and psychological health. Yet, dehydration is seldom recognized for what it is. To depend upon a feeling of dryness in our mouths alone to indicate when water is needed is not an accurate measure of the body's need for hydration.

As a general rule, most adults require at least a half gallon (2l) of water per day to be properly hydrated. While this may appear to be an excessive amount, consider the quantity of water that occurs naturally in the body. Conservatively speaking, water comprises about 85 percent of brain tissue and about 75 percent of the rest of the tissues in the body. To maintain the proper balance of water in the cells, then, a half gallon doesn't seem disproportionate. Fruit juice may be substituted for a portion of this fluid intake but shouldn't exceed more than 10 percent of the total. For an adult weighing over 200 pounds (90kg), an additional 8-ounce (250ml) glass of water for every 10 pounds (4.5kg) over that 200 mark is necessary to prevent dehydration.

The signs of dehydration range from the mild and most common to the most severe which may require hospitalization. Headaches, poor concentration and memory, constipation, and urinary infections are just a few of the results of improper hydration. If you are prone to illness, catching every virus that circulates through the office, you can be sure you're not drinking enough water. Increased feelings of stress from deadlines, difficult colleagues, and challenging patients may be nothing more than a signal that your body is in need of rehydration. Dry mouth, bad breath, and a furry-feeling tongue are additional warning signs that your tissues are becoming depleted. At its most severe, dehydration appears in the form of poor facial skin color, decreased muscle tone, muscle cramps, sunken eyes, and a rapid heart rate combined with fast and shallow breathing. Additionally, lack of proper hydration may lead to increased feelings of anxiety and bouts of depression.

In his book *Your Body's Many Cries for Water* (2008), F. Batmanghelidj, MD claims that dehydration provokes the same physiological response as that experienced by a person who is fatigued or under stress. In other words, the "flight or fight" response that we all feel when we become anxious also occurs when our bodies are not regularly and properly hydrated. According to Dr. Batmanghelidj, once the body is in distress, the materials that the body uses for dangerous or emergency situations (vasopressin, endorphins, cortisone release factor, rennin-angiotensin, and prolactin in women) begin to absorb the body's water reserves. The "flight or fight" response increases in proportion to the depletion of the body's reserves of water. At the same time, the endorphins, for example, continue to soak up more and more of the body's precious water supply. Add to cellular dehydration an unreasonably burdensome schedule of patients to see or patients who are difficult to satisfy, and the level of stress and fatigue rises significantly for the health care professional. Prolonged and repetitive stress reduces the level of energy generated in the brain. This electrical energy is essential for good mental as well as physical health. The brain is unable to produce the natural opiates that occur in the body because the brain cells become dysfunctional as a result of dehydration. Without the production of these hormones, particularly hydrocortisone and chemicals such as dopamine and serotonin, our pain threshold is lowered, and stored energy and raw materials cannot be converted into the additional energy necessary to cope with the increase in outside pressures. Without the ability to cope with the elevated levels of stress, some degree of depression is inevitable.

Hydration, however, is not our only concern. Because your patients are using Qigong and Taiji exercises to rid their bodies of toxins, you should make them aware of the importance of flushing these toxins thoroughly so that they will not remain trapped in the meridians or the juncture points where the meridians come together. If your patients are not limited in the quantity of fluids they can safely absorb, recommend that they keep a glass or bottle of water handy. At the end of each section, they might want to drink a few sips of water. If, at any time during your session, a patient indicates that he or she is particularly thirsty, fatigued, or furry-mouthed, stop the session and give that person time to drink enough water to feel comfortable again.

If you have patients who complain that they are urinating more often because of the increased intake of water and if no other medical condition is present, remind them that they may be flushing more toxins than usual.

Bear in mind, also, that if they have a history of not drinking much water, their bodies will need time to adjust to the sudden increase in fluids. Once they adapt to the new routine, the frequency of urination should reduce naturally.

Final reminders and suggestions

Now that you have reached the end of the book, you will have at least scanned through it and perhaps practiced some of the exercises. Repetition is the key to knowing and understanding these exercises so that the movements will flow and you will be able to lead your patients easily from one exercise to another. Check your patients periodically to be sure they are performing the exercises slowly and thoughtfully, with particular attention to their postures and breathing, and make certain that they are alternating between contracting and relaxing to avoid overuse of any set of muscles.

Posture is essential to the success of these exercise sessions. Proper posture is described at the beginning of each section but it is important to re-check frequently how your patients are sitting—for example, if they've begun to hunch over or if they've moved away from the back of their chairs. While it is natural and healthful to have a slight curve in the back when we're standing or lying down, you will want your patients to have their backs flat against the back of their chairs during most of these exercises to allow the *qi* to flow more easily through the meridians to and from the *dan tians*. Their feet should be flat on the floor, shoulder-width apart, their backs against the back of their chairs, hips tucked slightly under so that their backs are perfectly straight, shoulders rolled forward slightly. There are exceptions to this posture—for example, during *Flower Bud Opens*—so read the instructions carefully before you start your patients on each exercise.

Remember that, for most of these exercises, your patients will be using post-birth breathing—that is, expanding the diaphragm when breathing in and tightening it when they exhale. Pre-birth breathing is used for *Centering Qi* only, unless otherwise noted. In general, your patients' movements should be timed with their breaths: the deeper the breath, the slower the movement. Taking slow, deep breaths is one way to ensure that they won't rush through the exercises. Ideally, your patients will learn to time their movements with their breathing. As their breathing becomes deeper and slower, their movements will become more controlled and more effective.

How beneficial each session is depends not only on posture and breathing but also on the balance your patients are able to maintain between the *yin* and *yang* movements of each exercise. *Yin* refers to relaxed movements and *yang* to those times when muscles are tensed. To put it another way, your patients are in a state of *yin* when they are breathing in and their arms or legs are close to their bodies; *yang* occurs when they move their limbs away from the body and expel the air from the lungs. It is essential that there be an equal number of *yin* or very relaxed and preparatory movements offset by an equal number of *yang* or tense-muscled, strong movements. In this way, your patients' muscles will receive the strengthening they need but there will be no strain and no injuries.

For the purpose of clarity, I have described *qi* in a previous chapter as a disc or ball. I also mentioned a possible visualization of the energy's action you might want to use as the "sparks" thrown off by the momentum of the spinning disc. The basis of Taiji is *non-action* and, for that reason, it is helpful if you encourage your patients to think of themselves purely as a bundle of bones without flesh or muscle. Though it may seem contradictory, while you are directing them to take action and they strive to achieve the desired result, they are doing so in a *non-active* way, without straining muscles and stressing the body.

Before starting any of these exercises, take the time to help your patients center their bodies, minds, and spirits so they can concentrate entirely on their breathing and the movement of *qi* through the meridians of their bodies. Encourage them to rid themselves of any fuzziness or memories of unpleasant dreams from the night before if you are working with them early in the morning. If you are leading these exercises later in the day, you will want to help your patients rid themselves of the irritations and stresses they may have experienced earlier in the day.

Begin to bring your patients' "whole selves" into balance by asking them to visualize a rapidly flowing body of water. Direct them to imagine those ripples and waves as their days or nights, with the accompanying ups and downs. Ask them to concentrate on this image as they calm the waves until the water is as clear and smooth as glass. When you think they are sufficiently relaxed and centered, begin the exercises you have chosen for your patients for that session.

Music and readings

Many of my students ask about the music I use in class. I have an online store that carries a wide variety of Taiji, Qigong, and Feng Shui music, as well as general music CDs for relaxation and meditation. Of course, I recommend shopping at my store! The web address is www.healingtaichi.com.

In the interests of full disclosure, however, I must admit that there are a great many other sites that also offer appropriate music selections. You can check these out for use in your sessions by entering any of the terms listed above in the "search" box of your browser.

If you are interested in learning more about Taiji and Qigong, take a look at the books listed in the bibliography at the end of this book. I recommend all of them to you for further study. The more you, the health care professional, know about these ancient healing arts, the deeper the level of healing you will be able to offer your patients.

Appendix A

ABBREVIATIONS OF MERIDIANS

Lu   Lung

LI   Large Intestine

Sp   Spleen

TW   Triple Warmer

St   Stomach

SI   Small Intestine

H   Heart

CV   Conception Vessel

K   Kidney

P   Pericardium

B   Bladder

GB   Gallbladder

Lv   Liver

GV   Governing Vessel

EX   Extra Point

Appendix B

LOCATIONS OF ACUPRESSURE POINTS

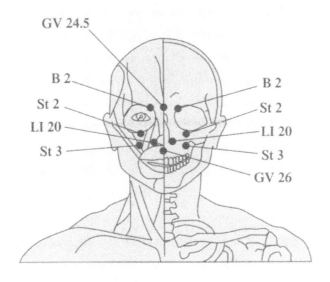

GV 24.5

B 2
St 2
LI 20
St 3

B 2
St 2
LI 20
St 3
GV 26

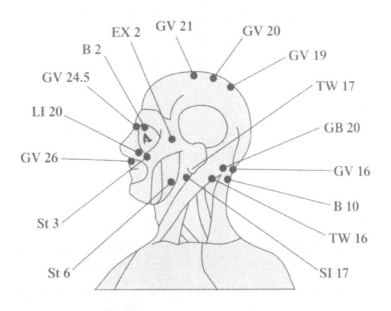

EX 2   GV 21   GV 20

B 2   GV 19

GV 24.5   TW 17

LI 20   GB 20

GV 26   GV 16

                            B 10

St 3   TW 16

St 6   SI 17

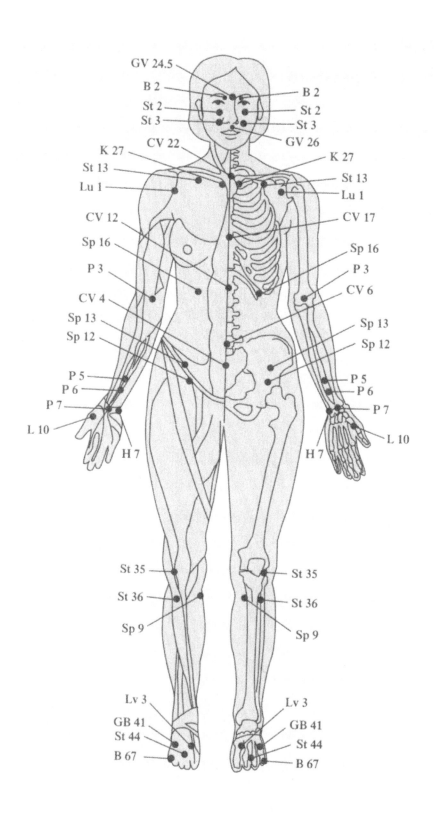

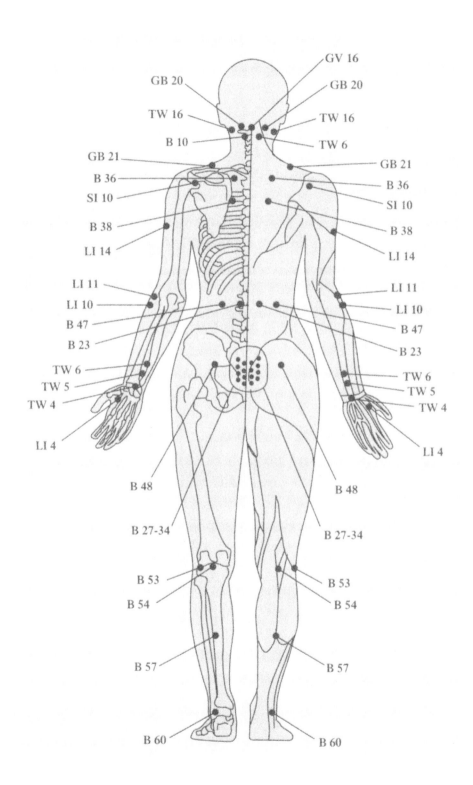

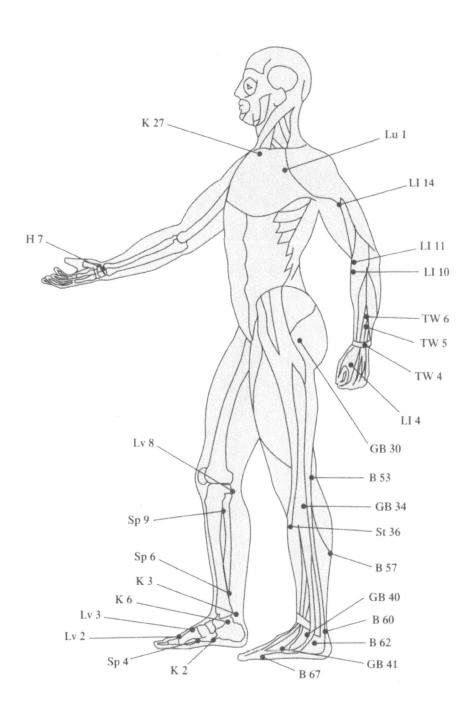

BIBLIOGRAPHY

Bankart, C.P. (1997) *Talking Cures*. Pacific Grove, CA: Brooks/Cole Publishing Company.

Batmanghelidj, F. (2008) *Your Body's Many Cries for Water*. Vienna, VA: Global Health Solutions.

Beling, J. (1999) "Twelve-month Tai Chi training in the elderly: Its effects on health fitness." *Physical Therapy 79*, 2, 208.

Birdsall, G. (1997) *The Feng Shui Companion*. Rochester, VT: Destiny Books.

Capra, F. (1983) *The Turning Point*. New York, NY: Bantam Books.

Capra, F. (1991) *The Tao of Physics*. Boston, MA: Shambala Publications Inc.

Cerrato, P.L. (1999) "Tai Chi: A martial art turns therapeutic." *RN Journal 62*, 2, 59–60.

Chuckrow, R. (1998) *The Tai Chi Book*. Boston, MA: YMAA Publication Center.

Cleary, T. (1994) *The Tao Classics*. Boston, MA: Shambala Publications Inc.

Cohen, K.S. (1997) *The Way of Qigong*. New York, NY: The Ballantine Publishing Group.

Crompton, P. (1987) *The Tai Chi Workbook*. Boston, MA: Shambala Publications Inc.

Dalton, J.O. (1994) *Backward Down the Path*. New York, NY: Avon Books.

Gach, M.R. (1990) *Acupressure's Potent Points*. New York, NY: Bantam Books.

Jou, Tsung Hwa (2001) *The Dao of Taijiquan to Rejuvenation*. Scottsdale, AZ: Taiji Foundation.

Kessenich, C.R. (1998) "Tai Chi as a method of fall prevention in the elderly." *Orthopaedic Nursing 17*, 4, 27–9.

Lam Kam Chuen (1999) *Chi Kung: The Way of Healing*. New York, NY: Broadway Books.

Lewis, D. (1997) *The Tao of Natural Breathing*. San Francisco, CA: Mountain Wind Publishing.

Liang, Shou-Yu (1996) *Tai Chi Chuan*. Roslindale, MA: YMAA Publication Center.

Liao, Waysun (1995) *The Essence of Tai Chi*. Boston, MA: Shambala Publications Inc.

Lin, D. (2006) *Tao Te Ching: Annotated and Explained*. Woodstock, VT: Skylight Paths.

LoBuono, C. and Pinkowish, M. (1999) "Moderate exercise, Tai Chi improves blood pressure in older adults." *Patient Care 33*, 18, 230.

Metzger, W. and Zhou, Peifang (1996) *Tai Chi Chuan and Qigong*. New York, NY: Sterling Publishing Co. Inc.

Ming-Dao, Deng (1992) *365 Tao*. New York, NY: Harper SanFrancisco.

Moran, E. and Master Joseph Yu (2002) *The Complete Idiot's Guide to the I Ching*. Indianapolis, IN: Alpha Books.

Needham, J. (1983) *Science and Civilisation in China: Vol. 5 Chemistry and Chemical Technology.* (Part 5 Spagyrical Discovery and Invention: Physiological Alchemy) Cambridge: Cambridge University Press.

Schorre, J. (1997) *How to Grasp the Bird's Tail If You Don't Speak Chinese.* Houston, TX: Arts of China Seminars.

Selye, H. (undated) "The Nature of Stress." Available at www.icnr.com/articles/the-nature-of-stress.html, accessed on 25 January 2012.

Wing, R.L. (1986) *The Tao of Power.* New York, NY: Doubleday.

Yang, Jwing-Ming (1999) *Taijiquan: Classical Yang Style.* Boston, MA: YMAA Publication Center.

INDEX

CPI Antony Rowe
Eastbourne, UK
June 20, 2023